Atlas of anatomical pathology of the gastrointestinal system of swine

For this English edition:

Atlas of anatomical pathology of the gastrointestinal system of swine

Plaza Antonio Beltrán Martínez nº 1, planta 8 - letra I
(Centro empresarial El Trovador)
50002 Zaragoza - Spain

First printing: May 2016

This book has been published originally in Spanish under the title:
Atlas de anatomía patológica gastrointestinal del cerdo

ISBN Spanish edition: 978-84-16315-79-6

Translation:
Owen Howard

ISBN: 978-84-16315-93-2
D.L.: Z 732-2016

Design, layout and printing:
Servet editorial - Grupo Asís Biomedia, S.L.
www.grupoasis.com
info@grupoasis.com

Warning:

Veterinary science is constantly evolving, as are pharmacology and the other sciences. Inevitably, it is therefore the responsibility of the veterinary surgeon to determine and verify the dosage, the method of administration, the duration of treatment and any possible contraindications to the treatments given to each individual patient, based on his or her professional experience. Neither the publisher nor the author can be held liable for any damage or harm caused to people, animals or properties resulting from the correct or incorrect application of the information contained in this book.

Atlas of anatomical pathology of the gastrointestinal system of swine

Serafín Gómez Cabrera

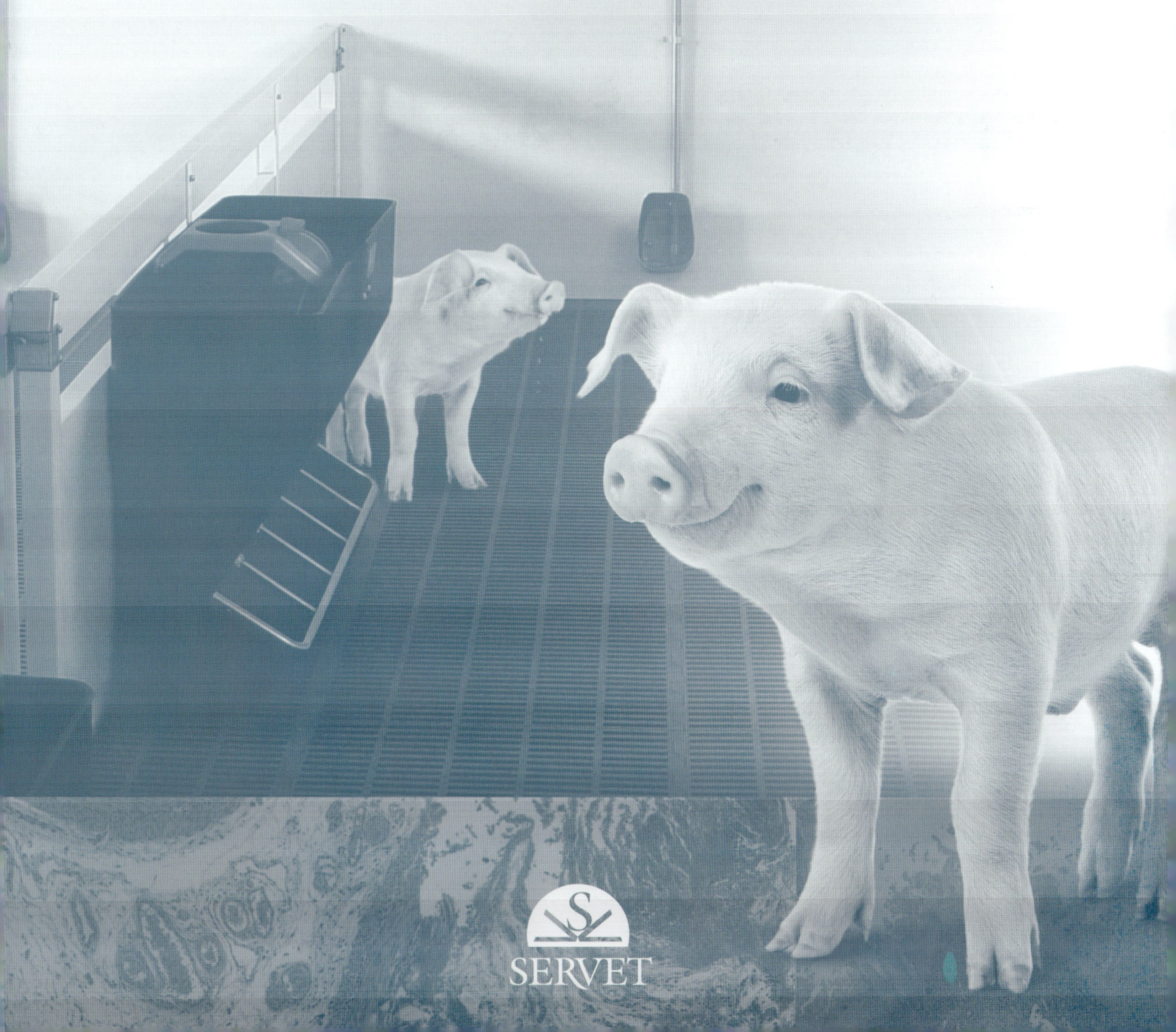

SERVET

The author

Serafín Gómez Cabrera

Bachelor in Veterinary Science from the University of Cordoba and PhD in Veterinary Medicine from the University of Murcia. After several years of professional experience in the private sector as a specialist in swine pathology, the author is currently Professor of Histology and Anatomical Pathology at the Faculty of Veterinary Medicine of the University of Murcia, a diplomate of the *European College of Veterinary Pathologists*, and a staff member of the Anatomical Pathology Service of the Veterinary Hospital of the University of Murcia.

Preface

This work is a visual guide to recognising and interpreting lesions that develop during the course of various gastrointestinal processes in swine, including alterations of the peritoneum resulting from its anatomical relationship with the digestive organs. The scope of this atlas is not limited to disorders caused by biological agents, which are of great importance in digestive diseases of swine, and includes a variety of processes of distinct aetiological origins.

The atlas contains images of gross and microscopic lesions. These are designed to complement one another, as the description of any pathological process is incomplete without considering the underlying histopathological changes. In some cases examples of normal organs and tissues are provided for comparative purposes.

The main objective of this atlas is to contribute to the interpretation of pathological processes using the main associated changes as the basis for a diagnostic protocol. Each image is accompanied by a description of the most salient features, avoiding where possible the theoretical speculation characteristic of textbooks. The images are interspersed with commentary on the differential diagnosis, taking into account the age of the animal, the area affected, and type of response elicited.

Although non-exhaustive by definition, this atlas is of great relevance given the importance of gastrointestinal diseases of swine. Our understanding of these conditions can be greatly enhanced through the study of pathological anatomy.

The author

Table of contents

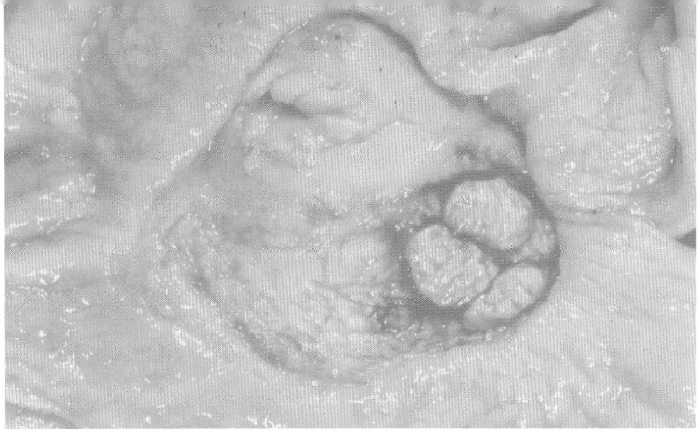

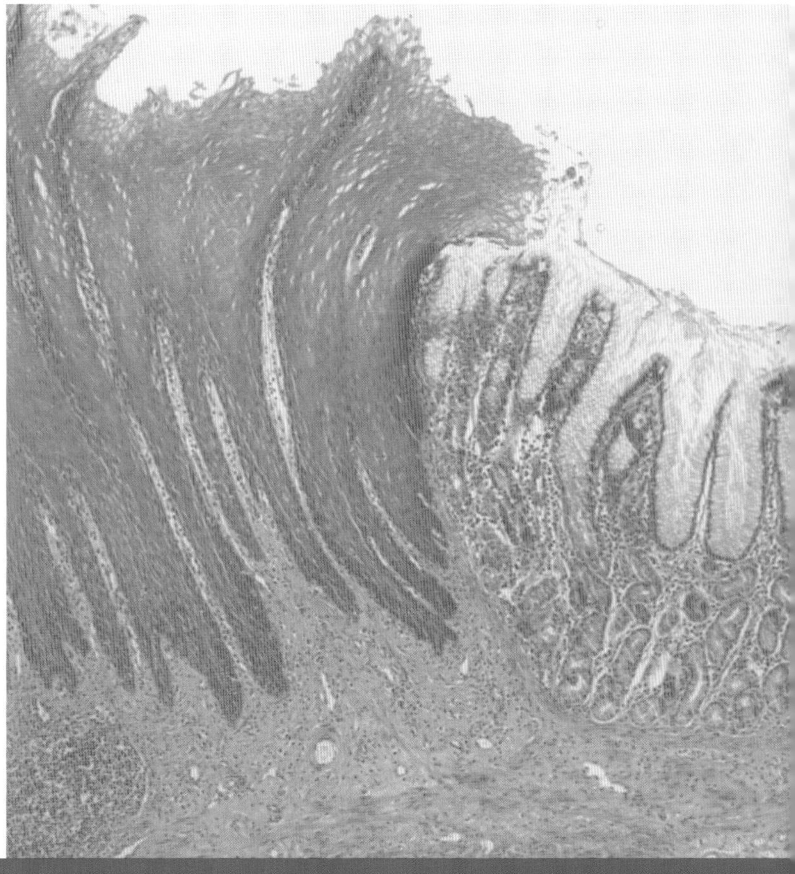

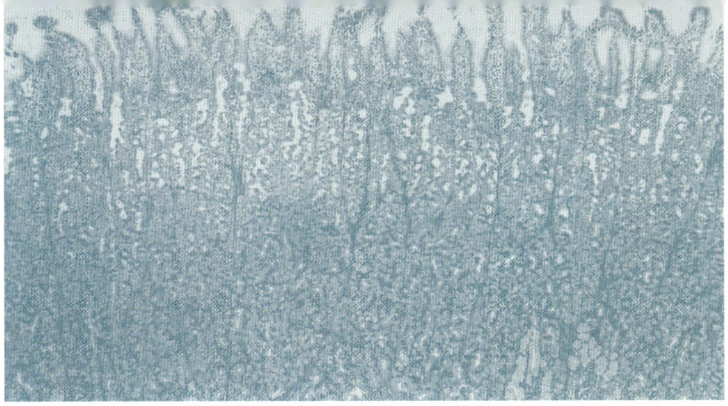

Stomach

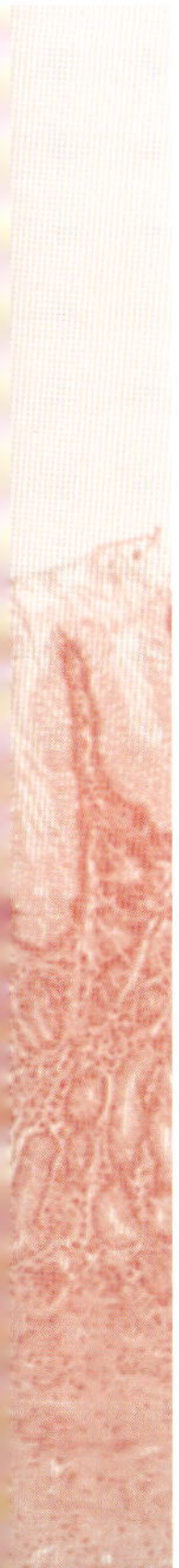

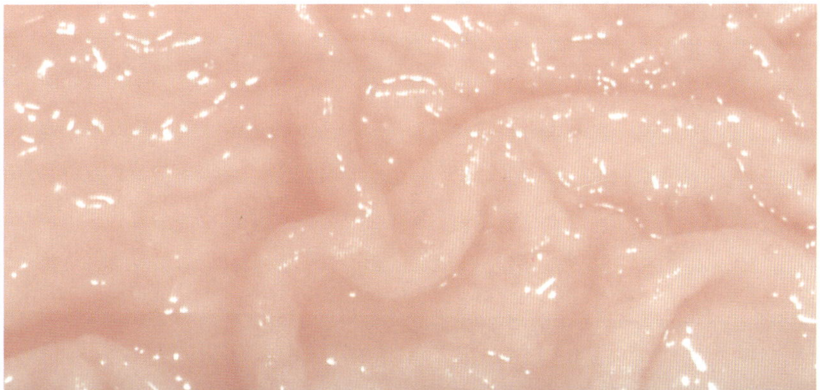

Postmortem changes

001A

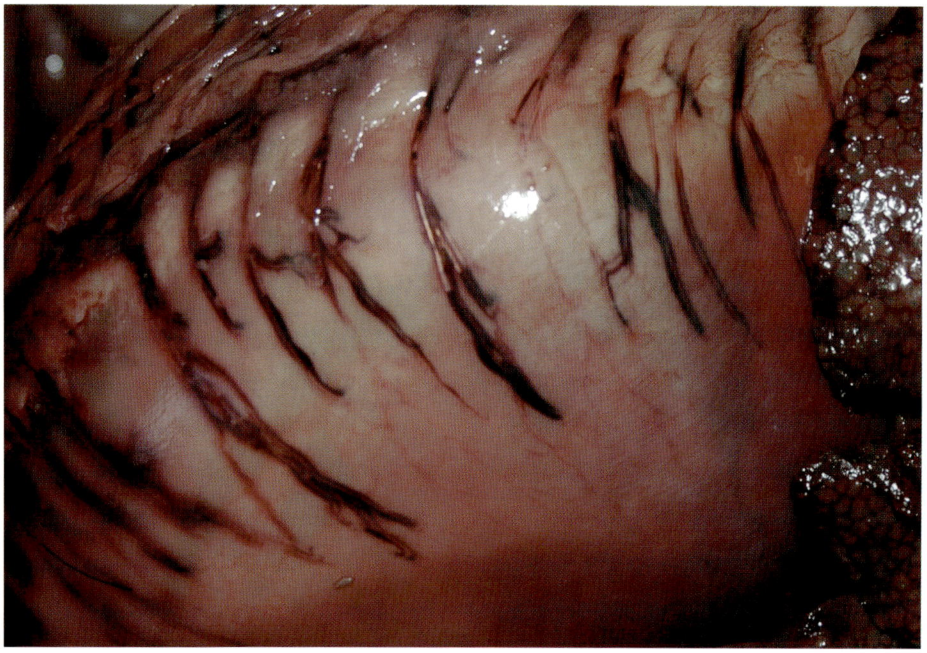

001B

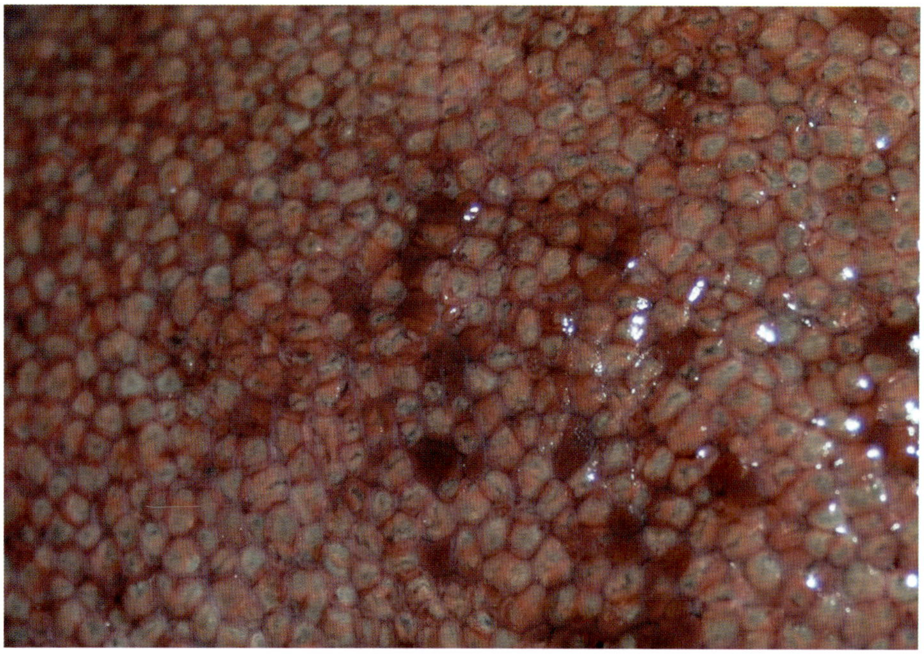

001A Haemoglobin imbibition.
Red colouration of the gastric serosa caused by diffusion of haemoglobin that has been degraded by autolysis. This effect is more pronounced throughout the vessels and areas that make contact with the liver.

001B Postmortem emphysema.
Liver surface with foamy aspect owing to the formation of bubbles due to bacterial activity.

Lesions of continuity

002

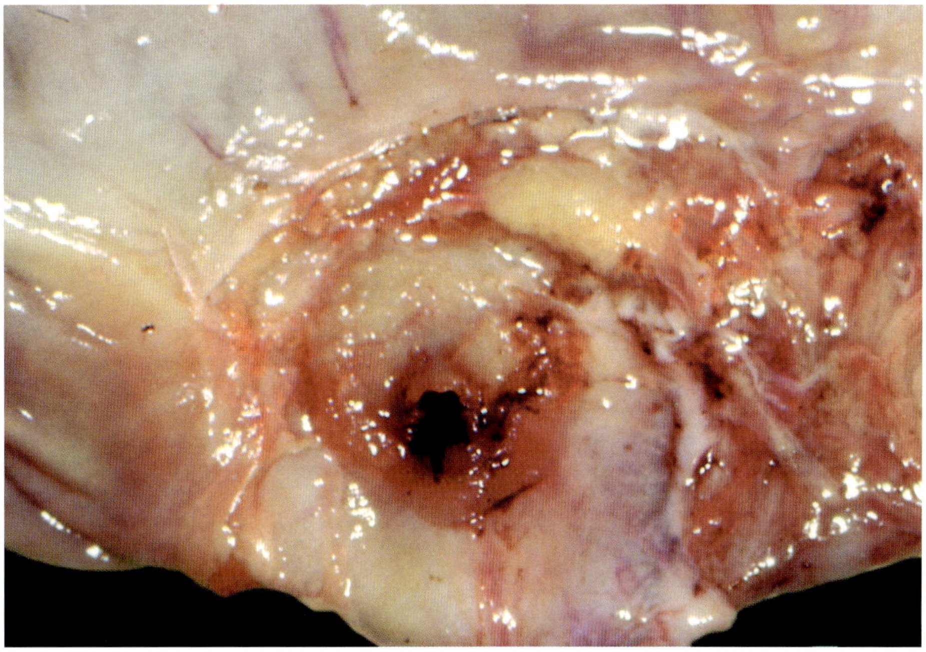

Gastric perforation can occur in different processes, such as ulcers, and can be caused by the corrosive action of aggressive chemicals, including iatrogenic agents.

003

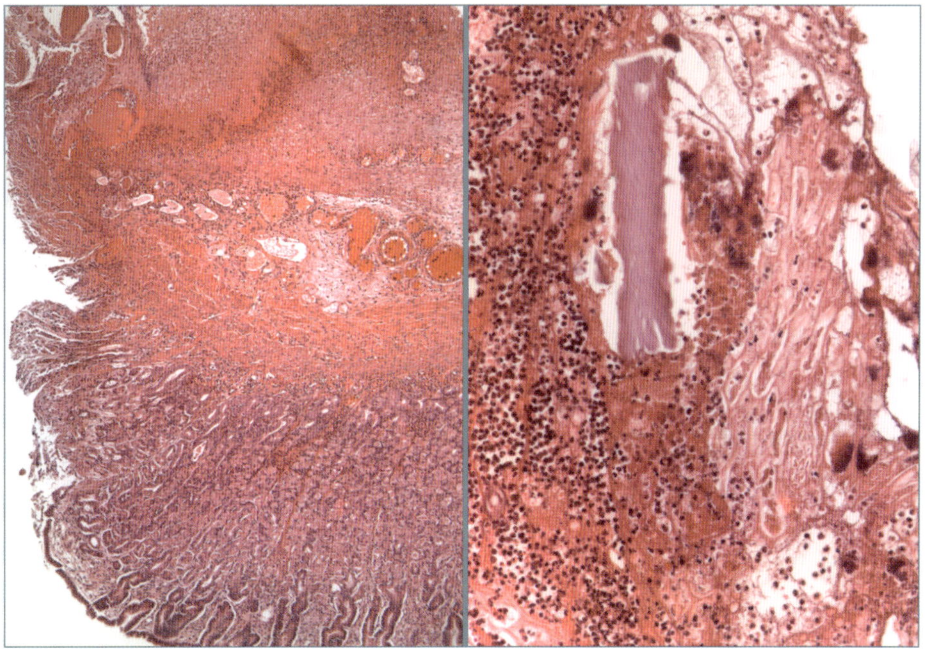

002 **Perforation.**
Loss of continuity of the gastric wall, affecting all layers, with reactive margins. Fattening pig.

003 **Perforation.**
All layers of the glandular stomach are affected by tissue destruction (left). Fibrinous exudate with leukocytes, bacteria, and plant debris in the serosa (right). Fattening pig. Haematoxylin-eosin (HE).

Erosions and ulcers

In this section it is important to distinguish between ulcerative processes of the non-glandular part of the stomach and those affecting the glandular regions.

004

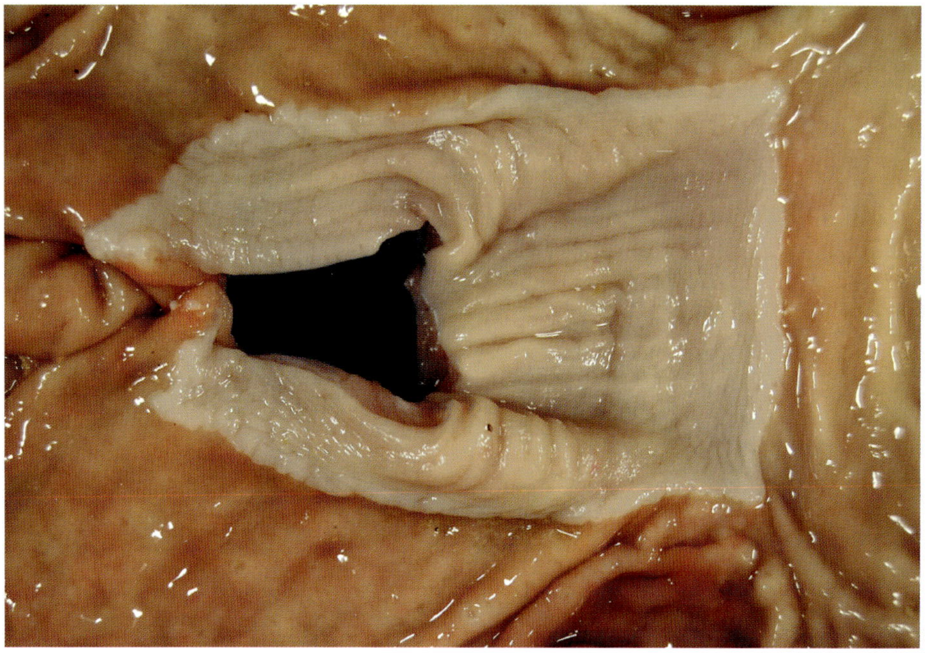

004
Porcine stomach.
Smooth, whitish aglandular mucosa with small, well-defined folds in the surrounding cardiac glandular region.

005

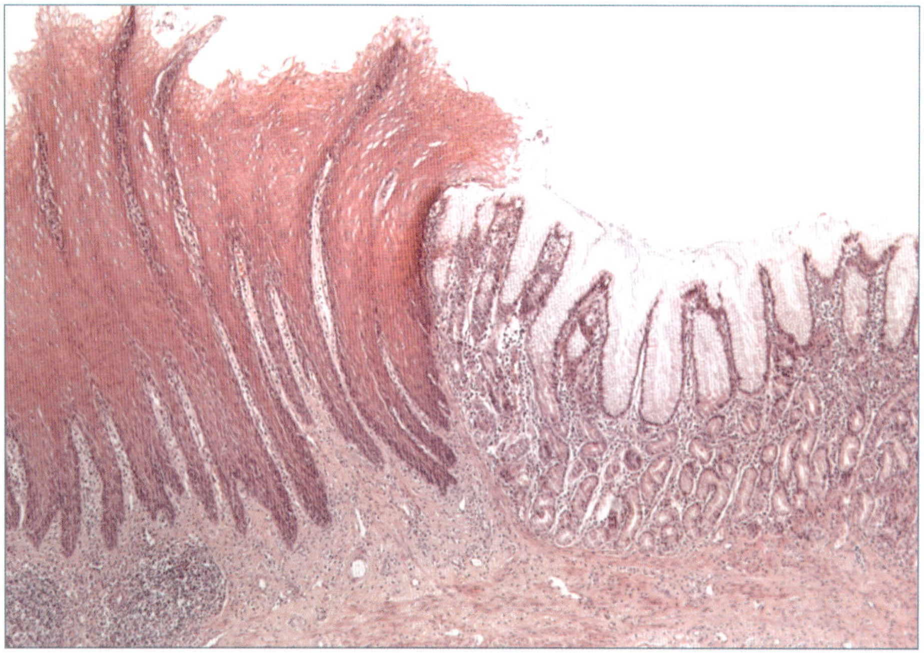

005
Porcine stomach.
Transition between the aglandular and glandular mucosa. Note the abrupt difference in the epithelia of the two regions. HE.

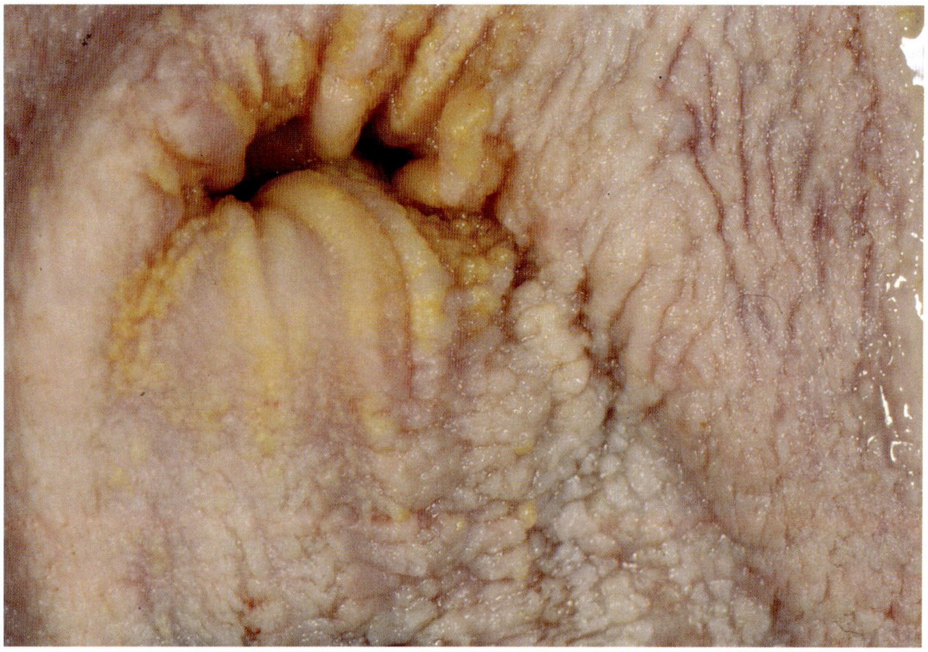

006A

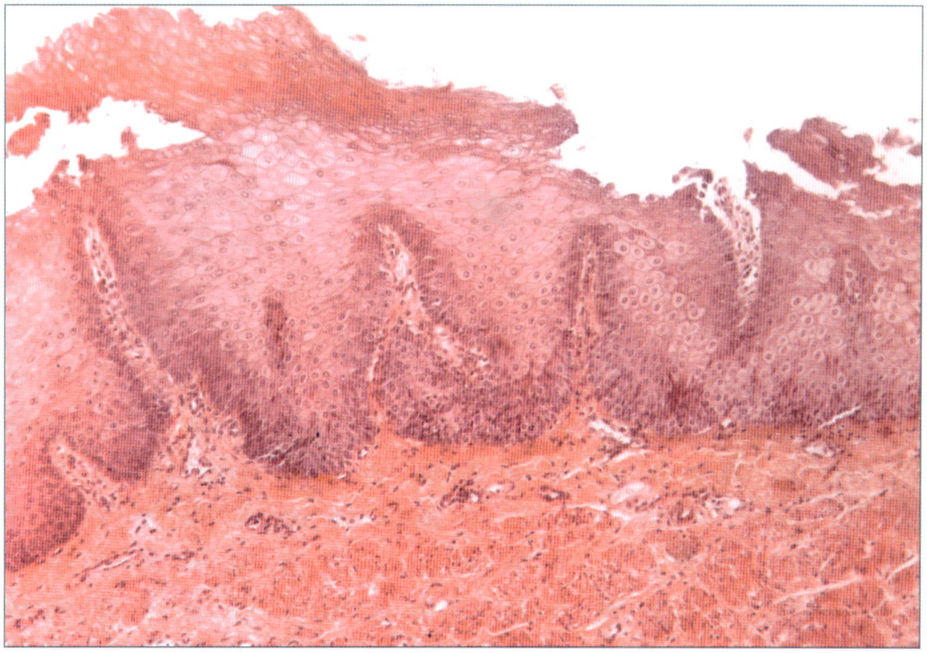

006B

006A Ulcerative changes.
Aglandular gastric mucosa displaying focal thickening of some folds, mild desquamation, and some biliary impregnation. Fattening pig.

006B Ulcerative changes.
Thickened, irregular epithelium with desquamation, erosion, and papillae in close proximity to the surface. HE.

007A

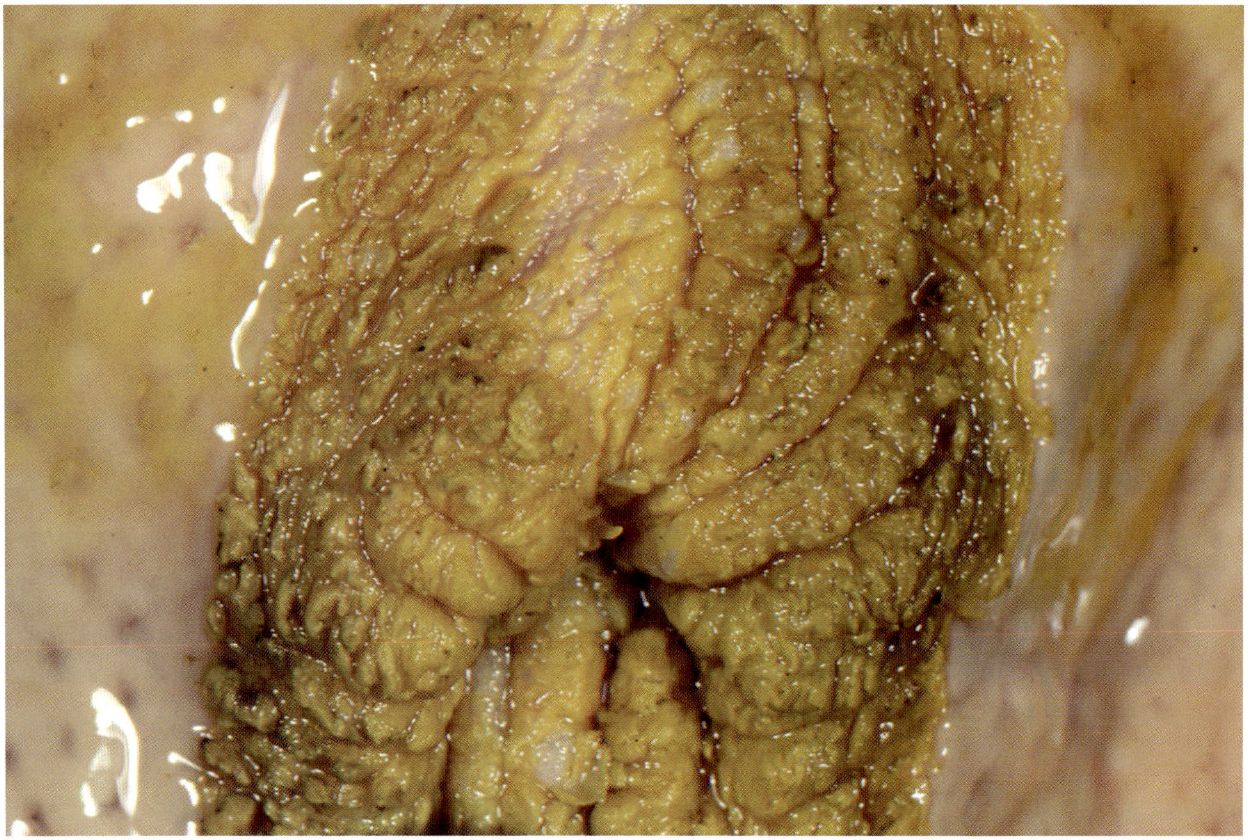

007A Parakeratosis.

Aglandular gastric mucosa is thickened, wrinkled, and fissured, with yellowish discolouration caused by biliary impregnation. Fattening pig.

007B

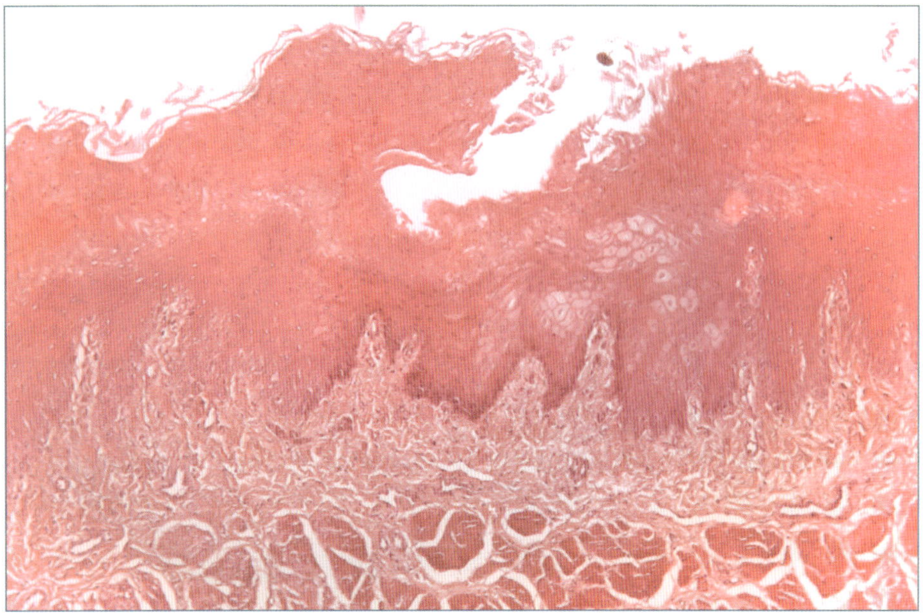

007B

Parakeratosis.

Epithelium of irregular thickness with desquamation, erosion, and irregular ridges. HE.

008A Ulcerative lesions.
Linear elevations of the aglandular gastric mucosa, which has a papillary, wrinkled, yellow-stained appearance. Fattening pig.

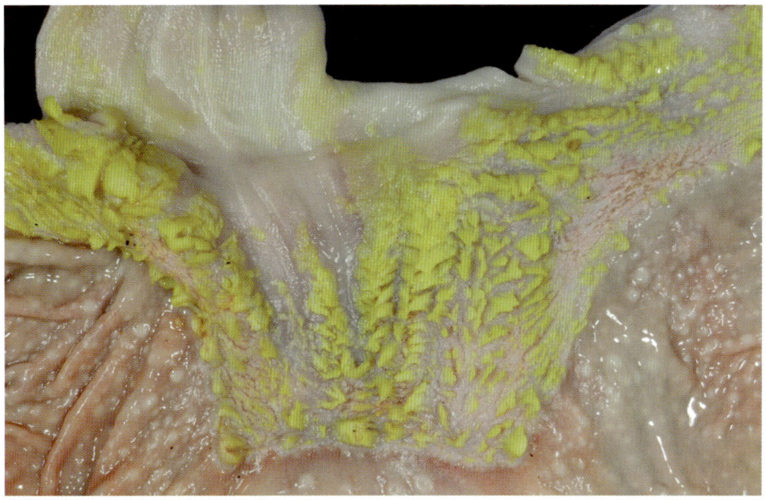

008A

008B Ulcerative lesions.
Irregularly thickened parakeratotic epithelium, with desquamation, erosion, and a fissure that extends to the lamina propria. HE.

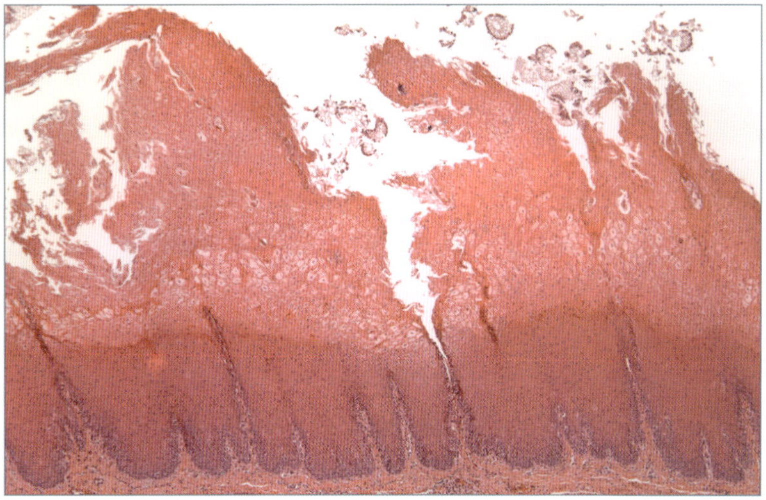

008B

008C Ulcerative lesions.
Hyperplastic and parakeratotic epithelium showing loss of continuity that extends to the underlying connective tissue. HE.

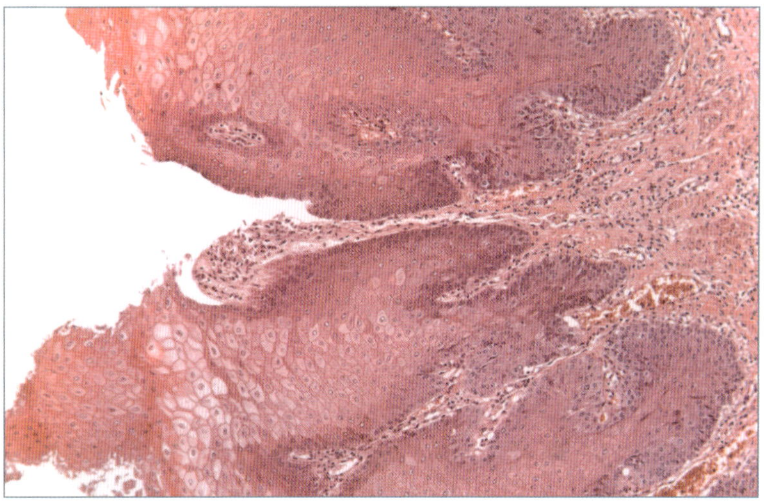

008C

009A

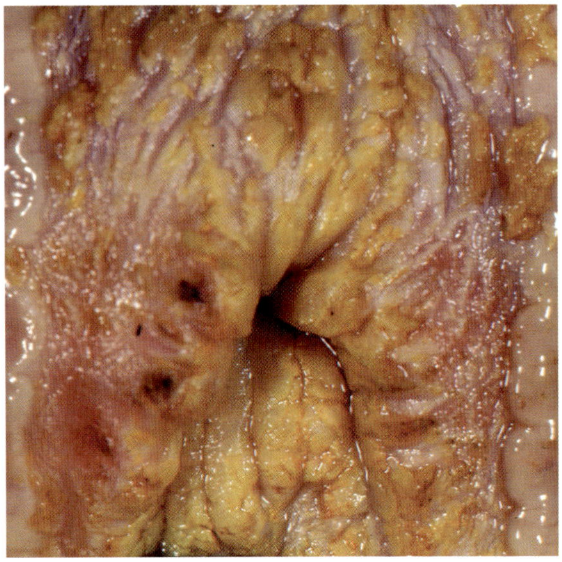

009B

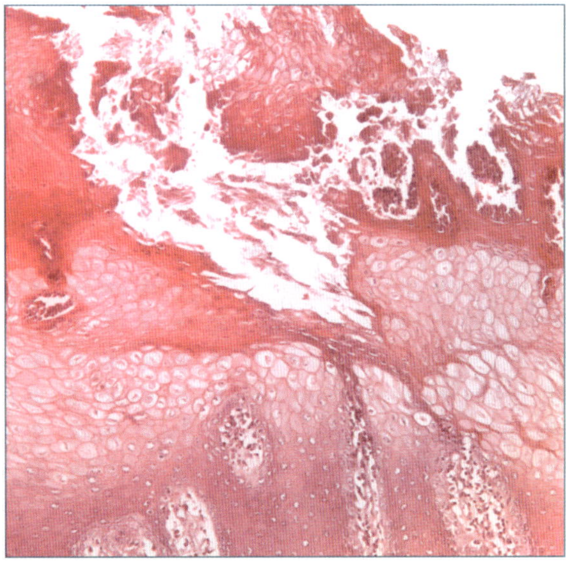

009C

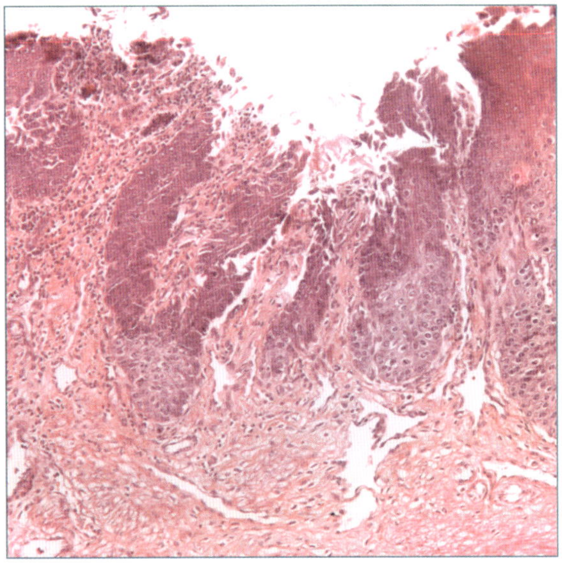

009D

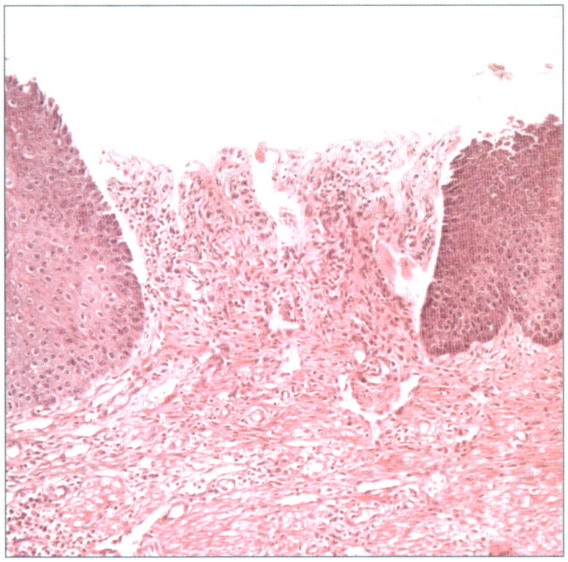

009 Progression of ulcerative gastric lesions in the aglandular region.

Wrinkled, fissured mucosa with linear erosions and areas of more extensive tissue loss with a reddish base (A). Parakeratotic thickening of the epithelium with desquamation and erosion (B). Narrow strips of tissue loss exposing the lamina propria (C). More extensive epithelial loss with exposure of connective tissue (D). Fattening pig.

Histopathological examination of these gastric lesions usually reveals the coexistence of different phases of the ulcerative process in the aglandular portion.

010 Ulcerative lesions.
Wrinkled, yellow-stained proliferations arranged radially around the cardia and distributed throughout the rest of the aglandular area, with multifocal tissue loss. Fattening pig.

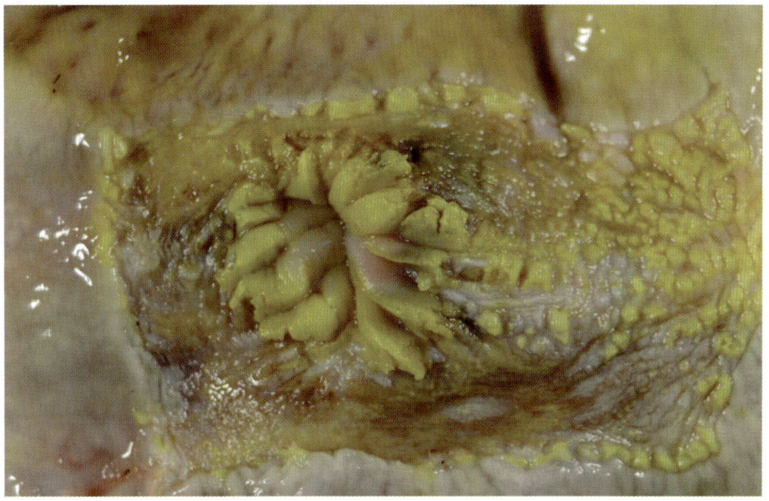
010

011A Gastric ulcer.
Thickened, wrinkled aglandular mucosa. The cardia is surrounded by a narrow band of excavation, with an off-white base and reddish foci. Fattening pig.

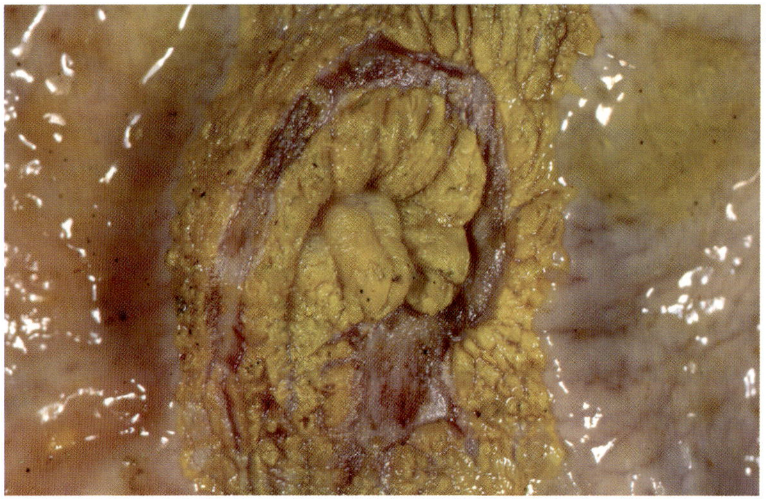
011A

011B Gastric ulcer.
Focal loss of mucosa exposing the connective tissue, next to an area in which the parakeratotic epithelium and elongated papillae are preserved. HE.

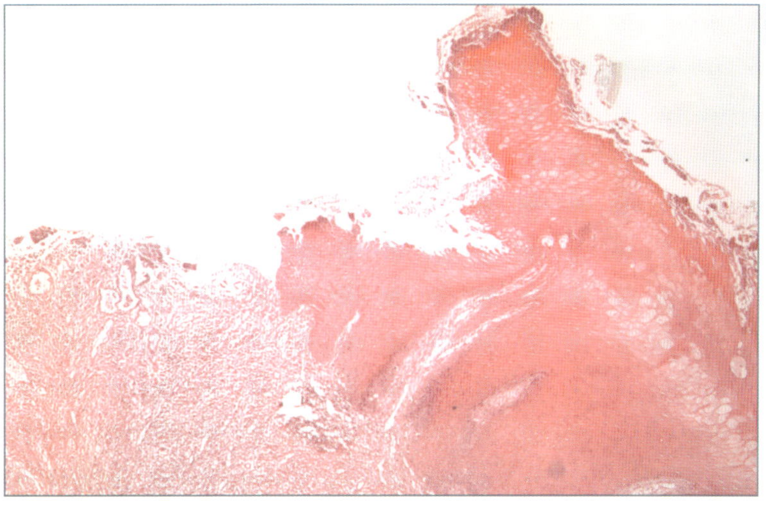
011B

012

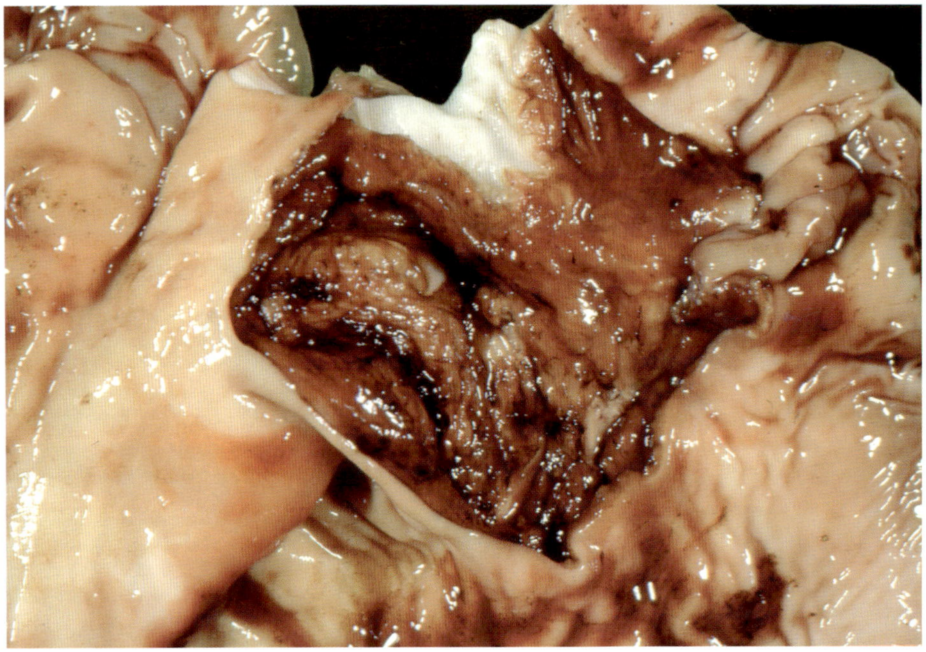

013

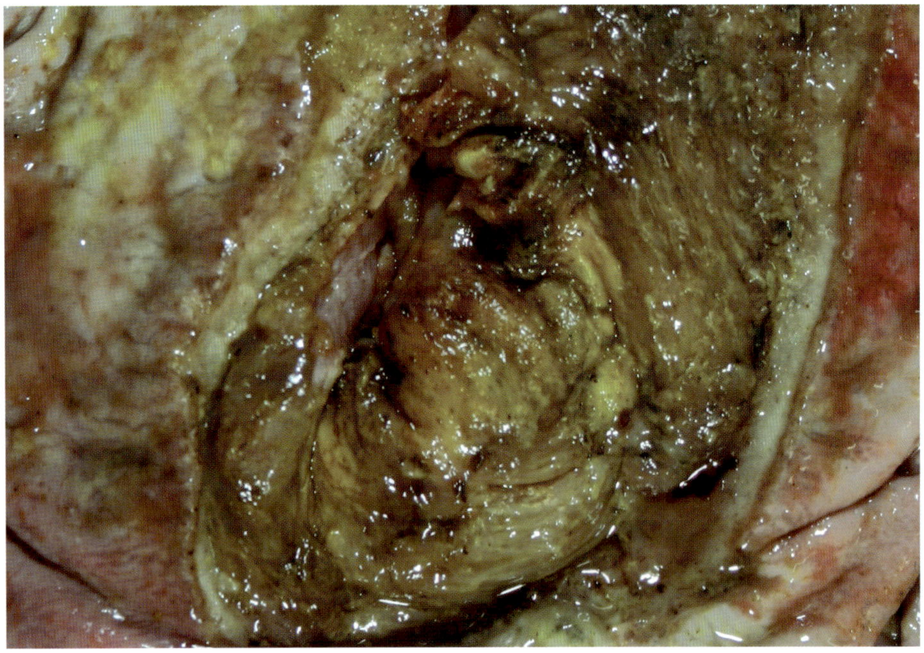

012 **Gastric ulcer.**
Excavating lesion with sharp margins, with destruction of the aglandular mucosa. The reddish base, with an uneven surface, contrasts with the white mucosa of the distal oesophagus. Fattening pig.

013 **Gastric ulcer.**
Extensive alteration of the aglandular portion, with foci of thickened mucosa and tissue loss of varying depths.
Breeding sow.

014A Chronic gastric ulcer.
Crateriform tissue loss in the aglandular portion, with irregular margins and thickened borders that protrude inwards. Fattening pig.

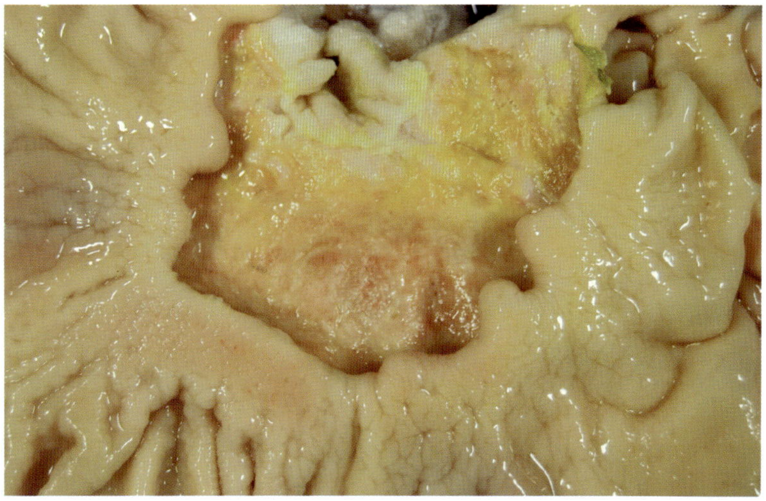

014A

014B Gastric ulcer.
Extensive mucosal loss with marginal conservation of the epithelium, which is covered by the mucosa of the adjacent glandular region. HE.

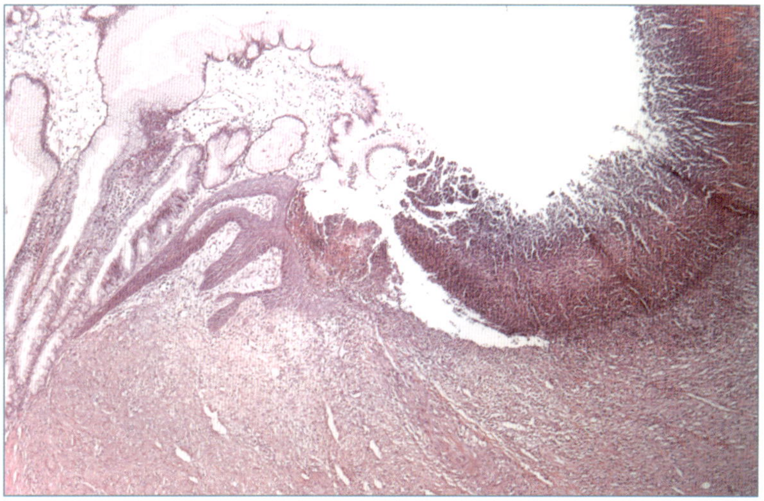

014B

014C Gastric ulcer.
Base of the ulcer consisting of a necrotic band over an area of granulation tissue and inflammatory cells. HE.

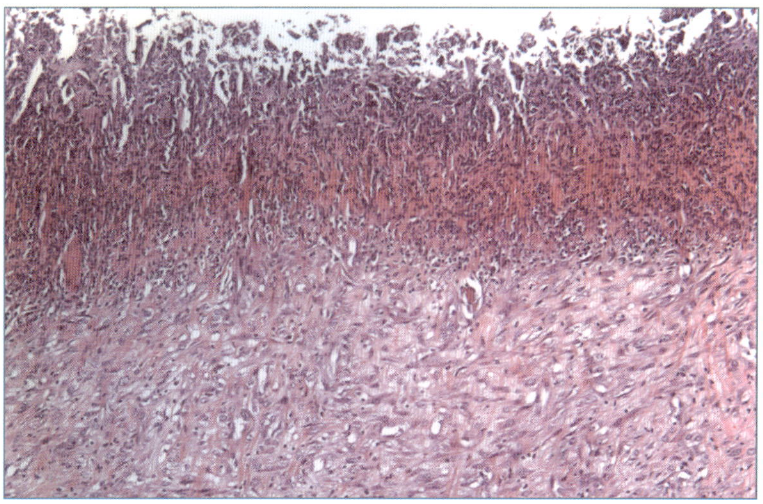

014C

015

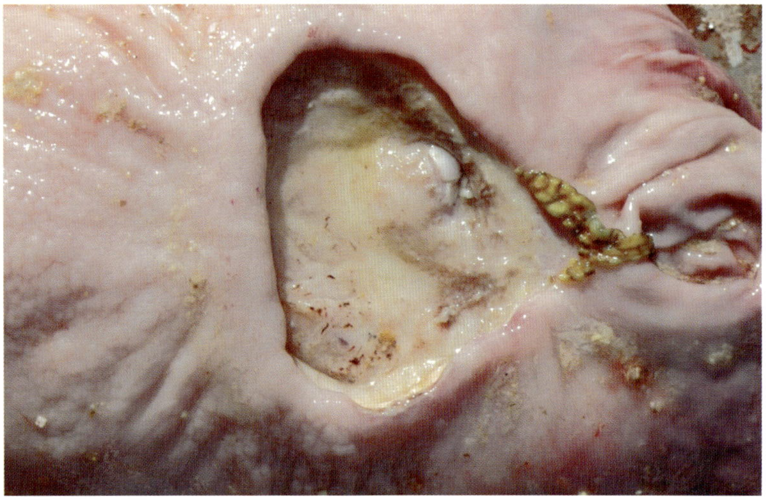

015 **Chronic gastric ulcer.** Crateriform lesion with prominent borders and retracted margins. The greyish, smooth-looking base lacks aglandular mucosa. Fattening pig.

016A

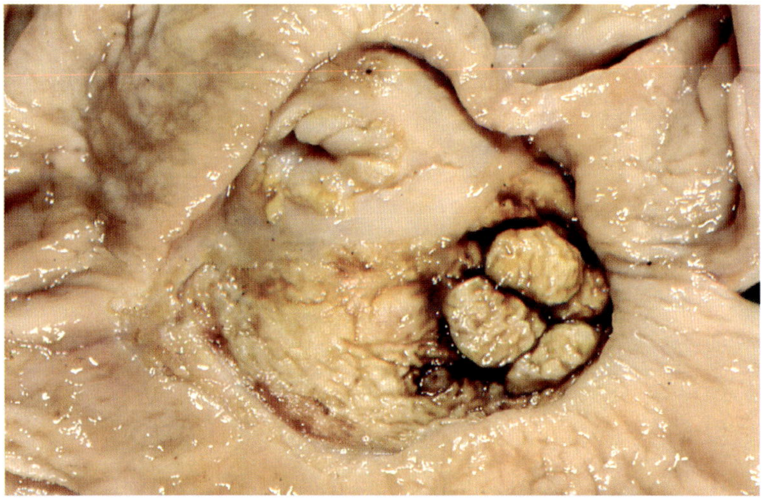

016A **Gastric lymphoid hyperplasia.** Whitish nodules on the base of a chronic ulcer in the aglandular region. Fattening pig.

016B

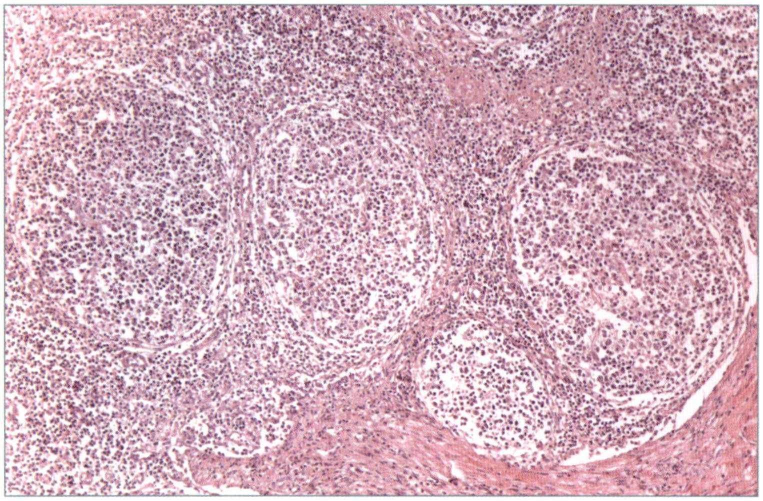

016B **Lymphoid hyperplasia.** Proliferation of mononuclear cells, which form lymphoid aggregates in the gastric submucosa. HE.

017 Scar retraction.

Sequela of a gastric ulcer with disappearance of most of the aglandular mucosa, of which wrinkled and yellowed epithelial remains persist. Fattening pig.

Gastric ulcers of the non-glandular portion are considered to be of multifactorial aetiology. Their development involves parakeratosis, erosion, and peptic (and in some cases perforating) necrosis. Gastric reflux can result in the spread of these lesions to the oesophagus.

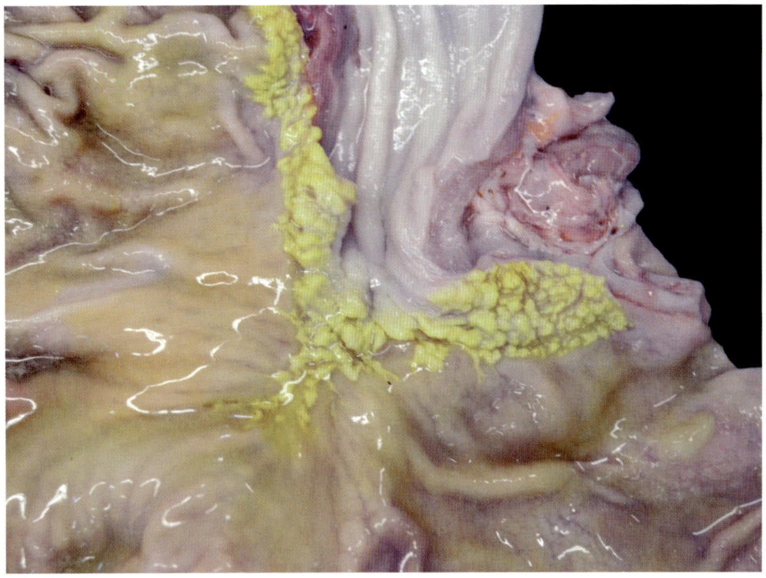

017

018A Gastric excavations.

Multifocal loss of the glandular mucosa of variable size, shape, and depth, corresponding to abrasions, erosions, and ulcers. Fattening pig.

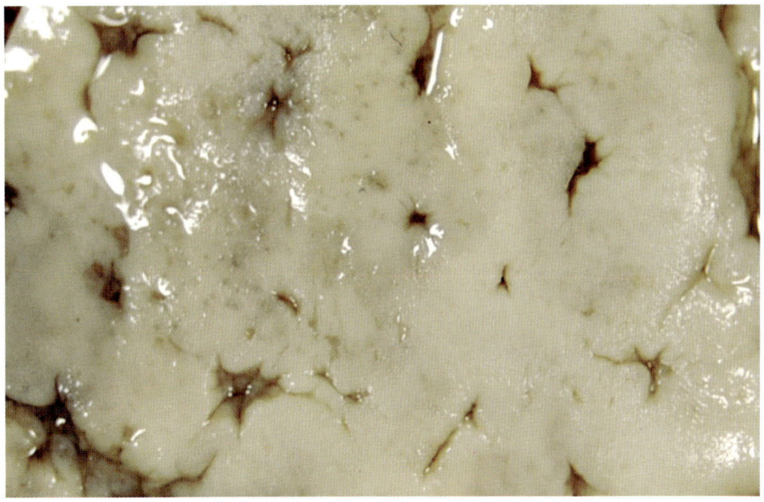

018A

018B Abrasion.

Tissue loss limited to the gastric surface epithelium. HE.

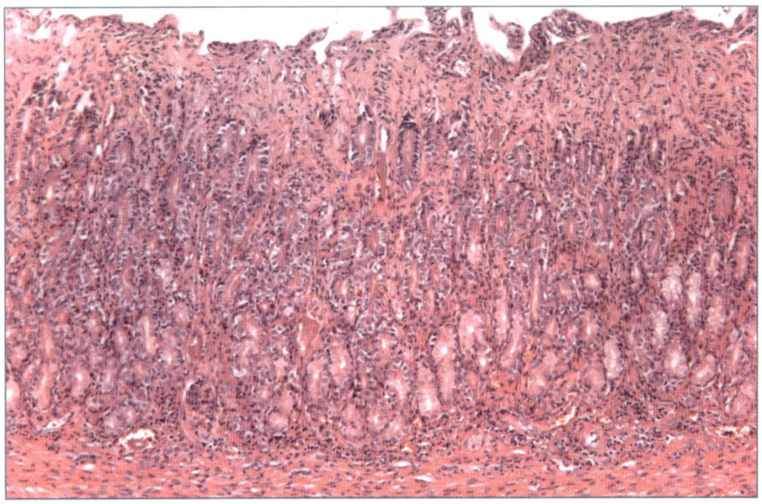

018B

018C

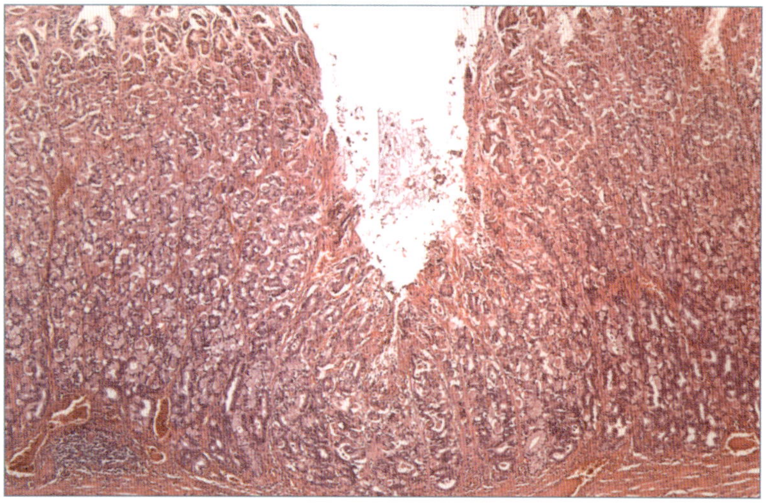

018C Erosion.
Focal tissue loss compromising part of the thickness of the gastric mucosa, with cellular and plant debris. HE.

019A

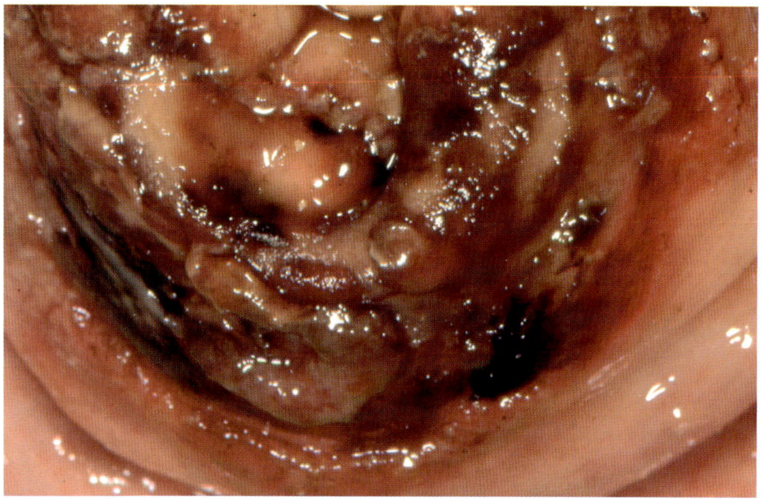

019A Erosive/ulcerative lesion.
Extensive focal loss of pyloric mucosa, with sharp borders and irregular reddish base with greyish deposits. Fattening pig.

019B

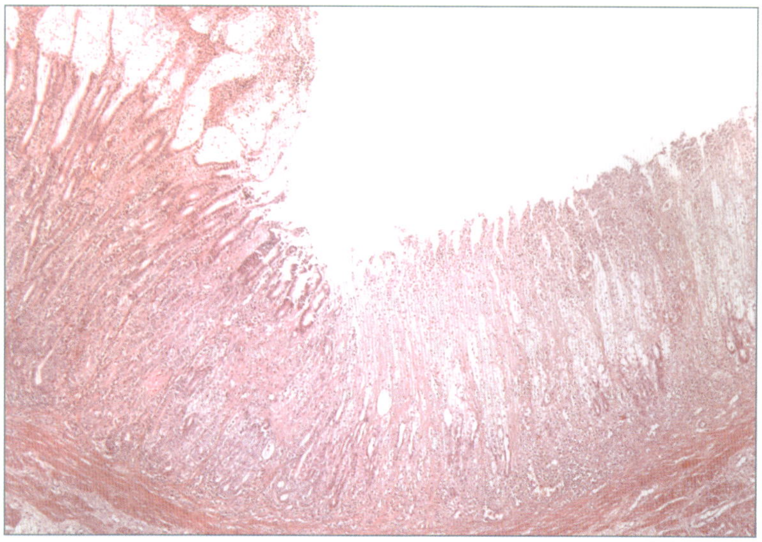

019B Necrosis.
Focus of altered mucosa, with conservation of the overall structure, that extends to the muscularis mucosae with loss of the superficial portion of the mucosa. HE.

020A Tissue loss.

Extensive focal lesion in the pyloric region, with reddish irregular base and greyish deposits. Fattening pig.

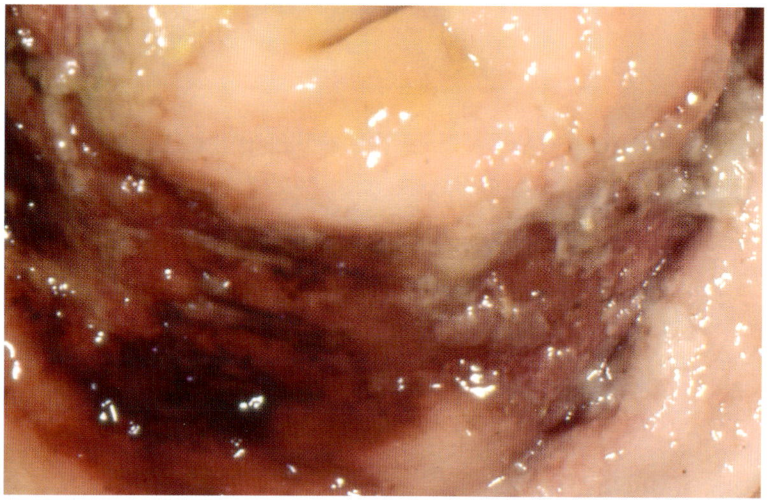

020A

020B Necrosis.

Mucosal alteration, with conservation of tissue layers, that extends down to the muscularis mucosae with superficial tissue detachment. HE.

These lesions caused by tissue loss are not considered primary inflammatory processes, but rather necrotic foci with variable exudative phenomena.

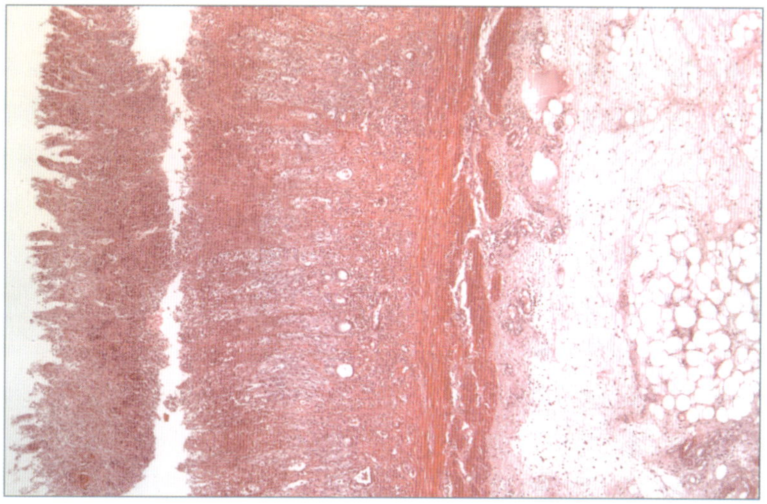

020B

021 Ulcerative lesions.

Confluent, sinuous excavation of the glandular gastric mucosa, consistent with erosion and ulceration.

The development of ulcers in the glandular region is associated with oral administration of NSAIDs, irritating compounds, systemic infections, parasites, and stress.

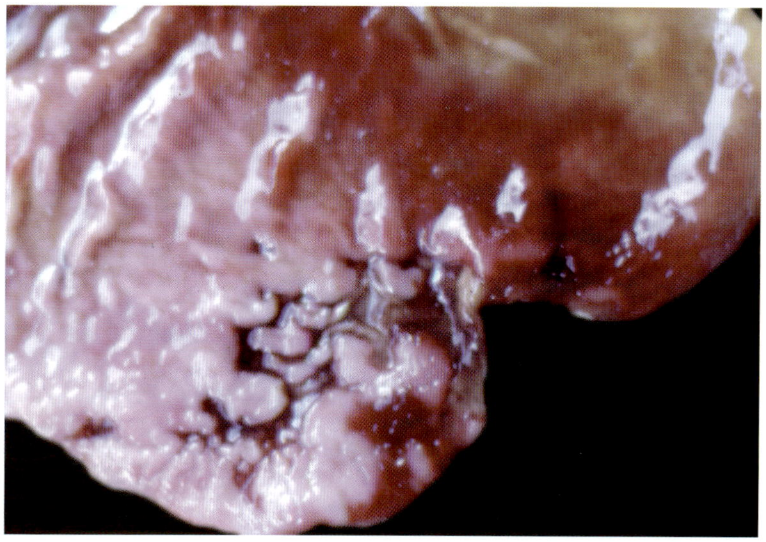

021

Circulatory disorders

022

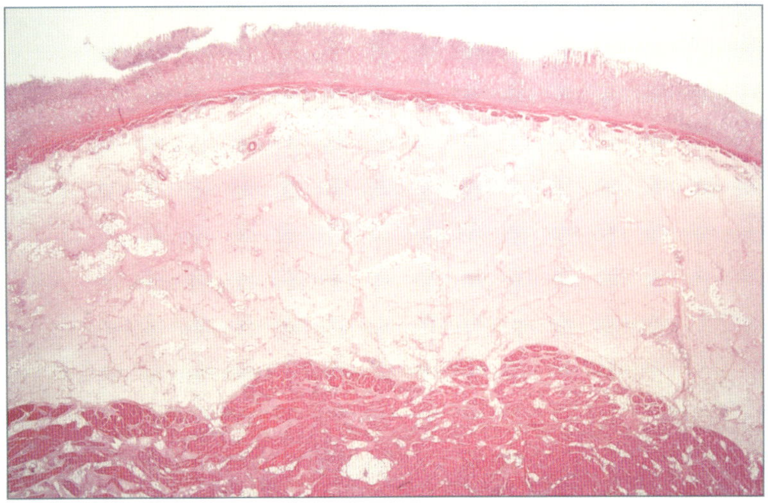

022 **Oedema.**
The widest, least stained, central band corresponds to the gastric submucosa, which has been thickened due to abnormal accumulation of fluid in the intercellular space. Fattening pig. HE.

023A

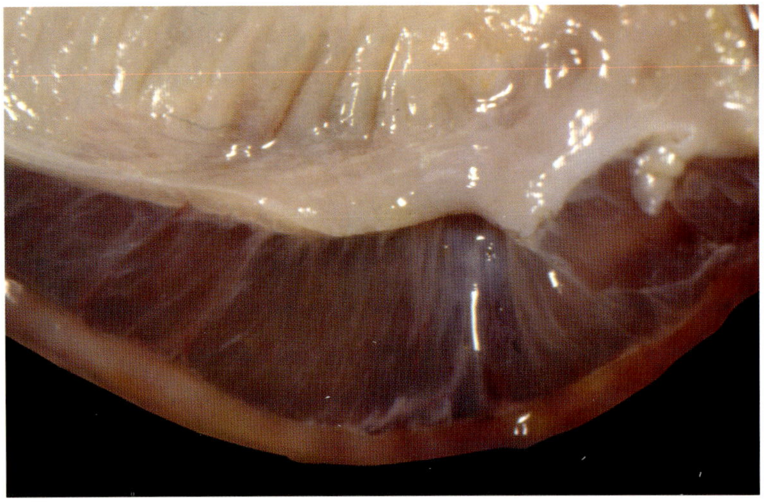

023A **Oedema.**
Surface of a section of the gastric wall, which has been thickened by a gelatinous band corresponding to the submucosa. Weaner pig.

023B

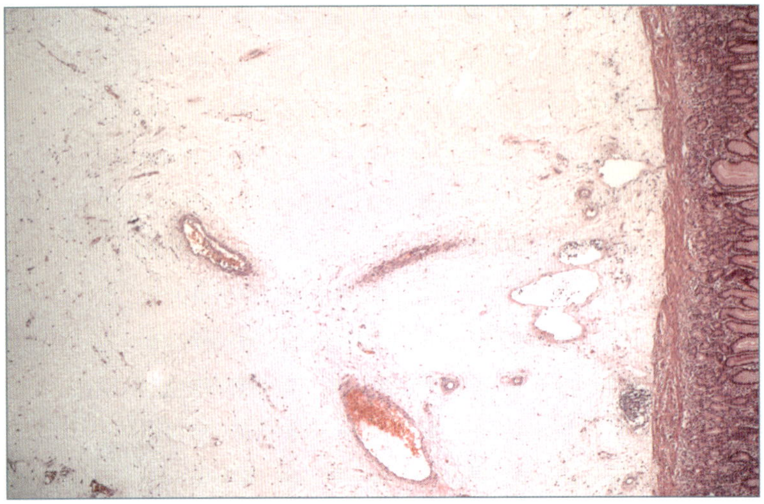

023B **Gastric oedema.**
Expansion of the submucosa caused by the accumulation of fluid between the tissue components. HE.

024A Oedema.

Area of gastric mucosa displaying turgid folds and a glassy appearance (left). Section of the gastric wall showing gelatinous thickening of the submucosa (right). Weaner pig.

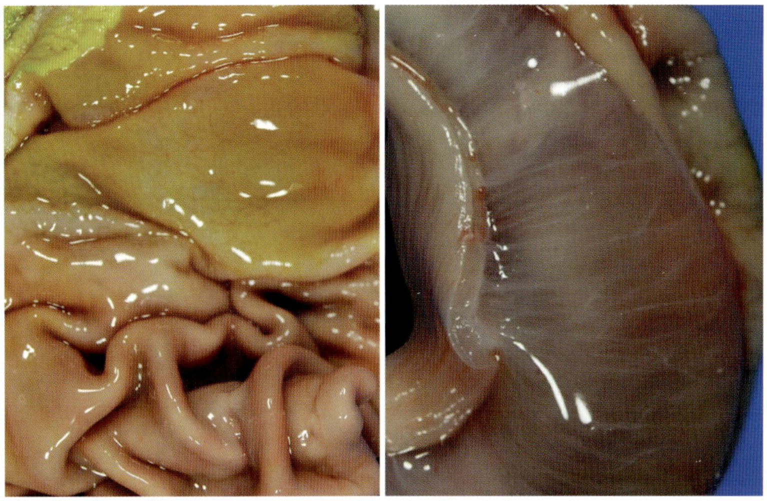

024A

024B Gastric oedema.

Enlarged submucosa with dissociation of tissue components due to abnormal accumulation of fluid in the intercellular space. HE.

> Gastric oedema is predominantly submucosal. This type of lesion is characteristic of oedema disease, but can also present in conjunction with other metabolic, circulatory, toxic, and inflammatory processes.

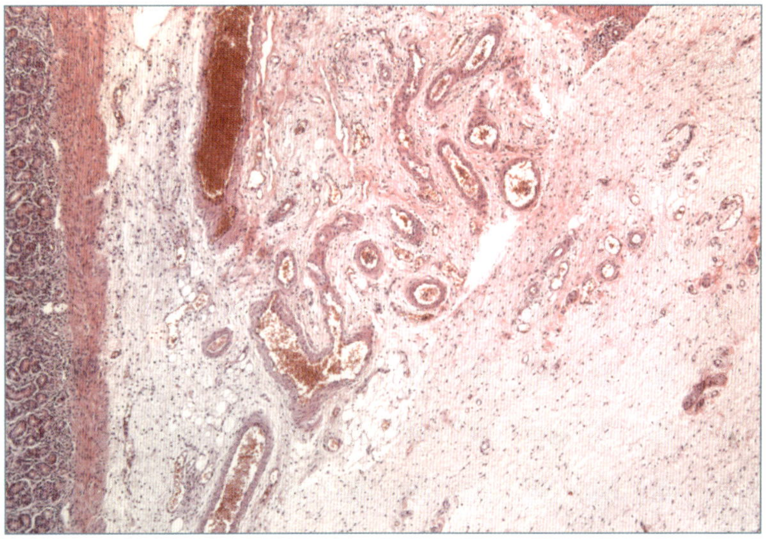

024B

025 Hyperaemia.

Focally extensive reddening of the gastric mucosa. Weaner pig.

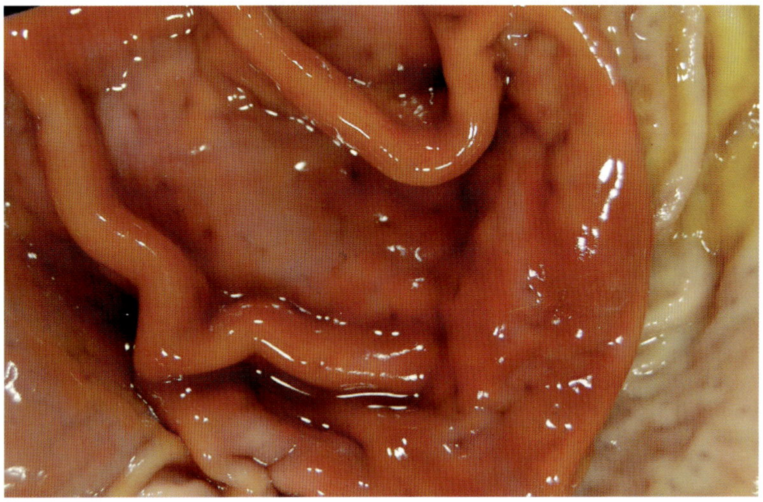

025

026

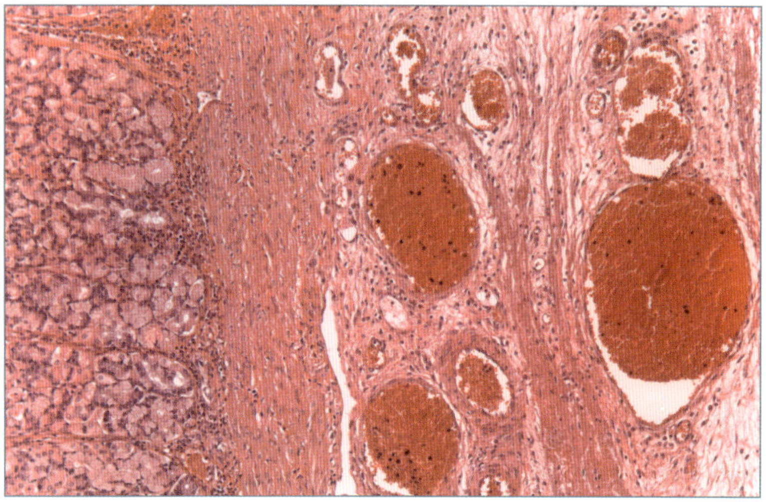

026 **Hyperaemia.**
Dilated, erythrocyte-filled blood vessels of the gastric wall. Fattening pig. HE.

027A

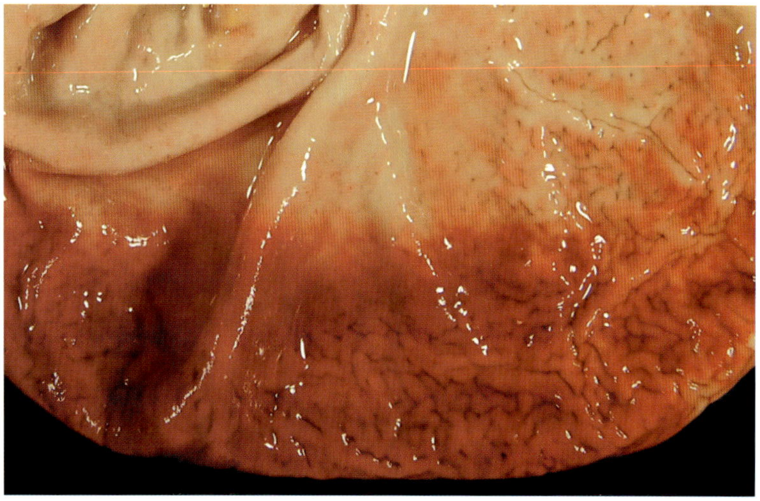

027A **Hyperaemia.**
Marked, focally extensive reddening of the gastric mucosa. Weaner pig.

027B

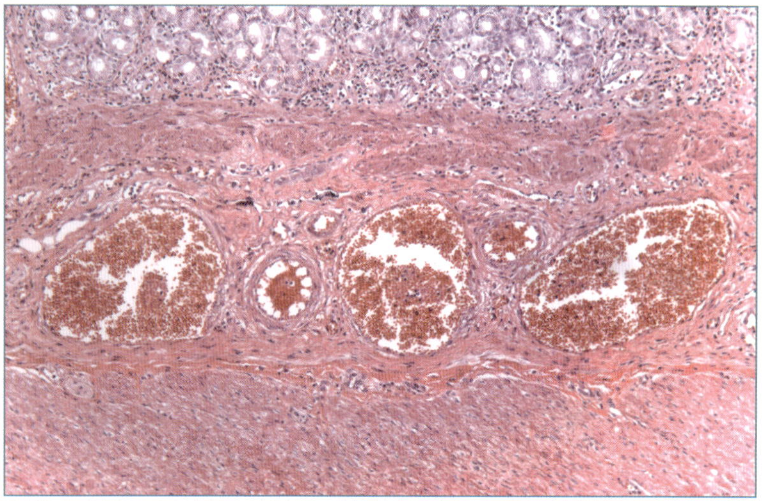

027B **Hyperaemia.**
Dilated, erythrocyte-filled blood vessels of the gastric wall. HE.

Active hyperaemia is physiological during digestion. The pathological form appears in acute gastritis of chemical, toxic, metabolic, or infectious aetiology. Passive hyperaemia is associated with portal hypertension and circulatory failure.

028A Gastric infarction.

Fundic mucosa with a marbled appearance displaying extensive dark red to blackish foci and dull grey areas. Fattening pig.

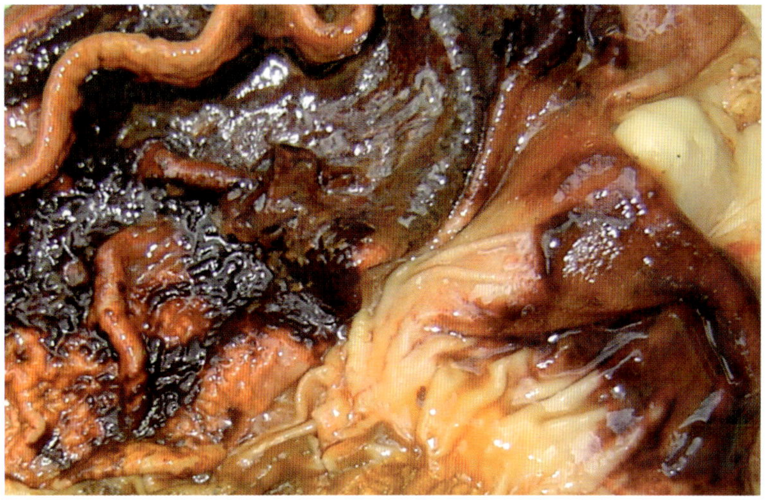
028A

028B Gastric infarction.

Superficial necrosis of the mucosa, with haemorrhage and thrombosis of the microvasculature. HE.

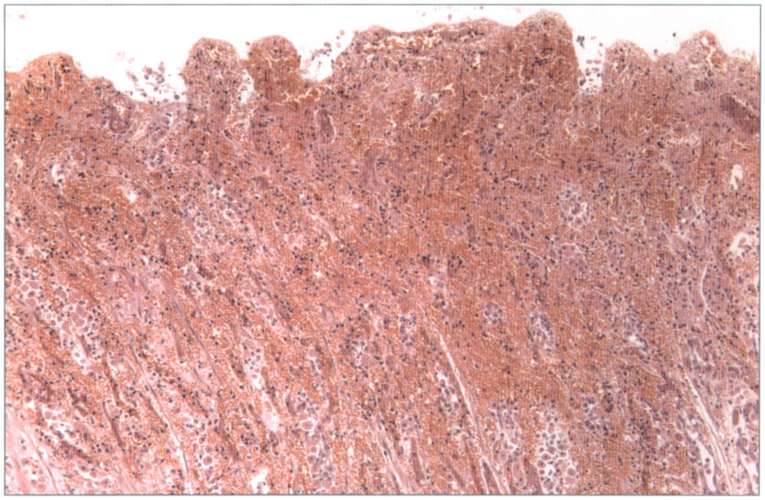
028B

Gastric infarction occurs in processes that present with endothelial damage, such as salmonellosis, colibacillosis, swine fever, erysipelas, dysentery, polyserositis, and mycotoxicosis.

029 Thrombosis.

Intravascular coagulation with parietal adherence of the vessels of the gastric submucosa. Fattening pig. HE.

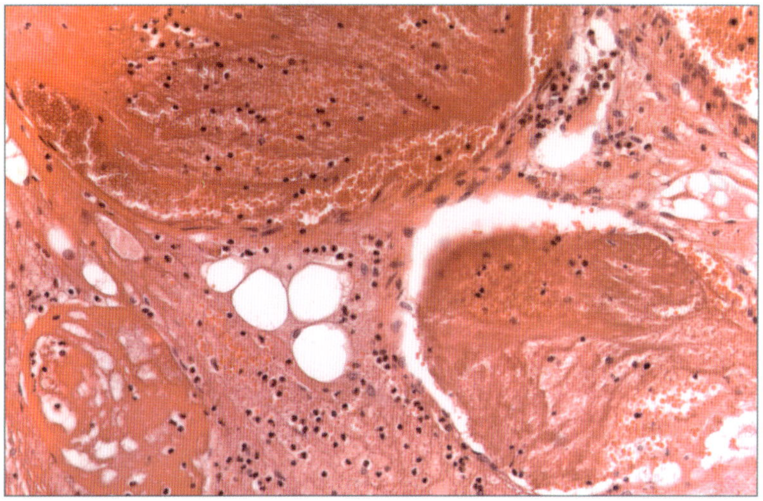
029

Inflammation

Many lesions of the stomach described as gastritis are in fact of a noninflammatory nature. The term should be reserved for cases that fulfil the histological criteria for gastric inflammation. Some denominations, despite their frequent use, are histopathologically imprecise.

030

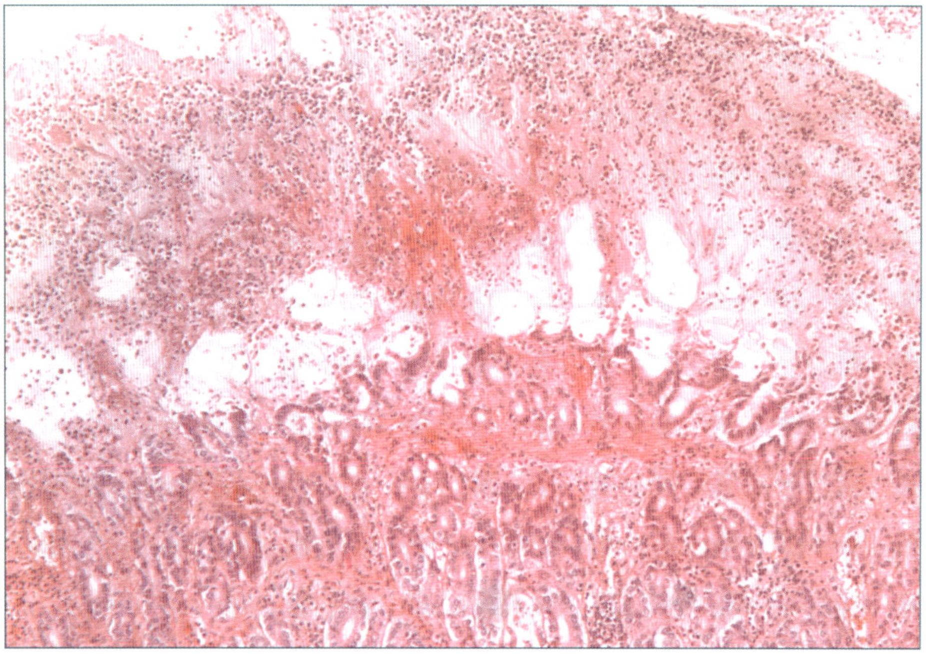

030
Fibrinous exudate.
Pseudomembrane formed by cell debris, fibrin, and leukocytes, with surface alteration of the gastric mucosa in an erosive-ulcerative lesion. HE.

031

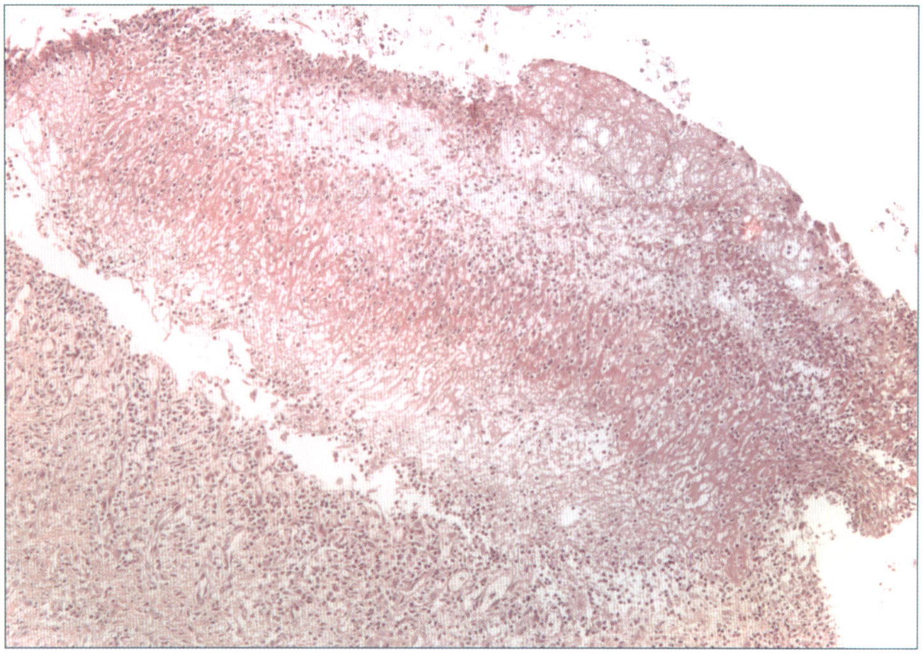

031
Fibrinous exudate.
The pseudomembrane, consisting of cell debris, fibrin, and leukocytes, sits on a necrotic focus of the gastric mucosa in an erosive-ulcerative lesion. HE.

032A

Chronic gastritis.
Thickened cardiac mucosa focally covered by adherent, yellowish-grey deposits. Replacement sow.

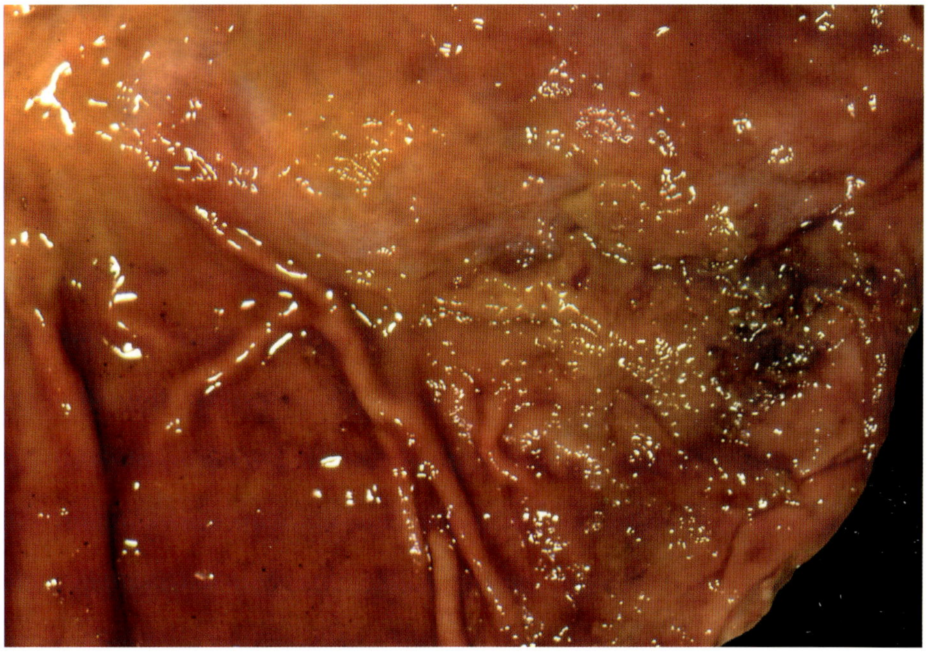

032A

032B

Chronic gastritis.
Enlargement of the lamina propria caused by a predominantly lymphoplasmacytic inflammatory cell infiltrate. Exudate consisting of mucus and sloughed cells. HE. Spiral bacteria in the exudate (right). Warthin-Starry (WS).

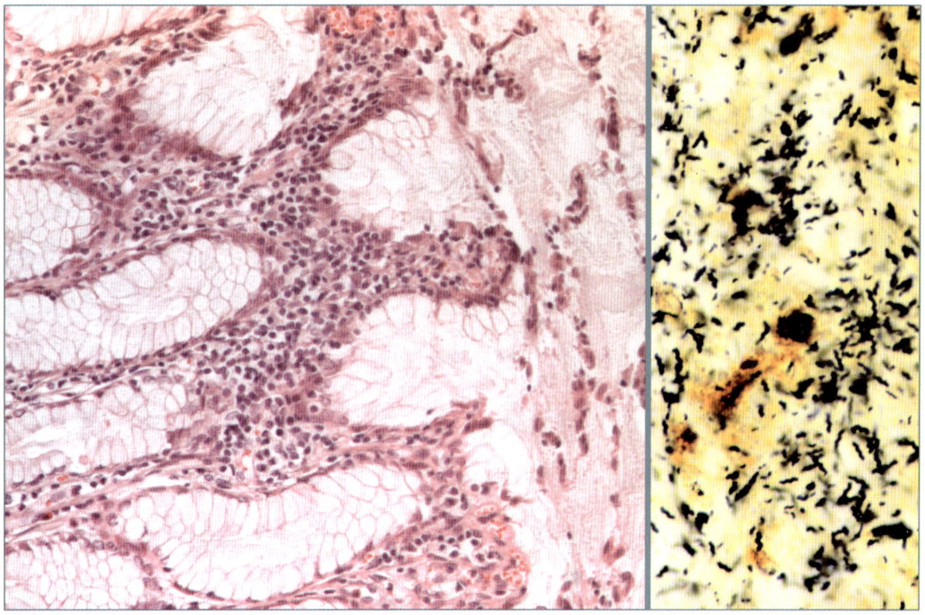

032B

Acute catarrhal gastritis is associated with infections such as colibacillosis and transmissible gastroenteritis. Non-erosive pseudomembranous gastritis is generally caused by biological processes, including fungal infections, swine fever, and salmonellosis. Chronic nonproliferative gastritis can be the manifestation of local processes or of syndromes involving multiple organ failure.

033

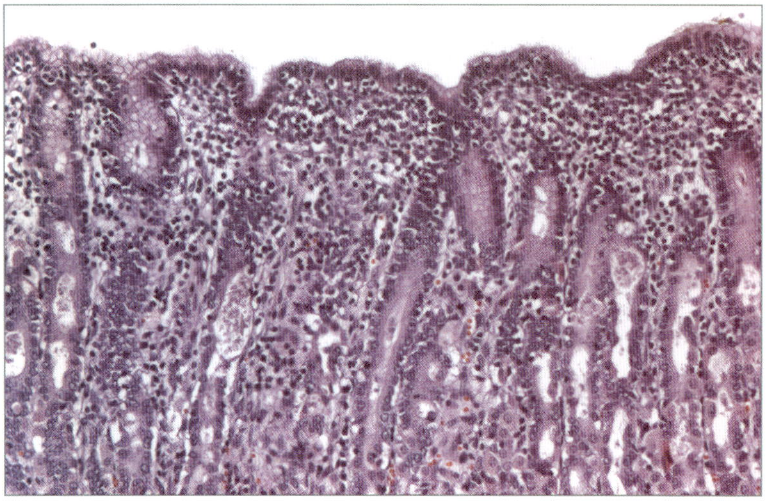

033 **Chronic superficial gastritis.**
Dense lymphocytic infiltrate in the distal third of the lamina propria with some disorganisation of the glands. This inflammatory process is not usually associated with characteristic gross alterations. Weaner pig. HE.

034A

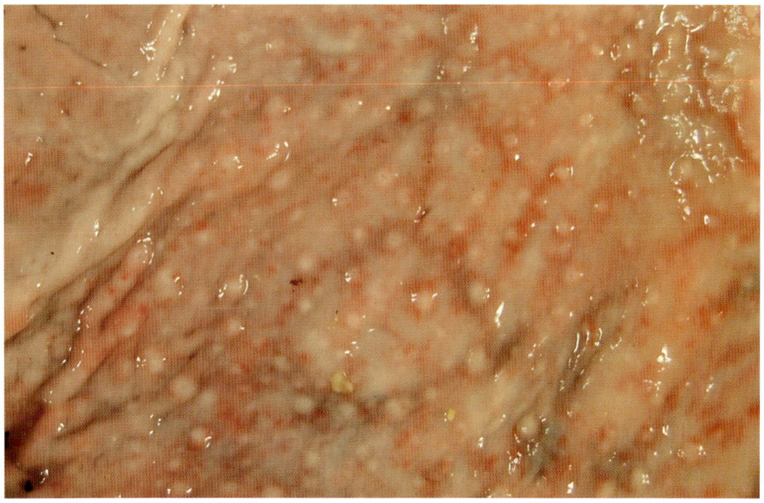

034A **Follicular lymphoid hyperplasia.**
Mucosa of the glandular stomach dotted with whitish nodules. Weaner pig.

034B

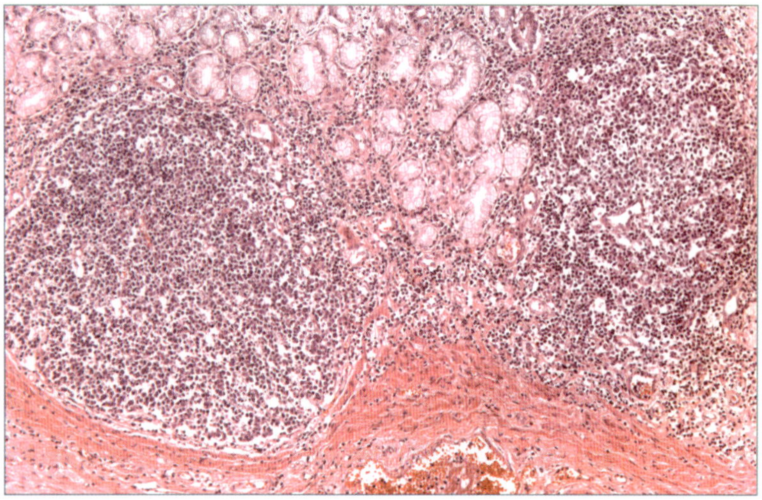

034B **Follicular lymphoid hyperplasia.**
Presence of enlarged lymphoid follicles with lymphocytic infiltration in the lamina propria of the gastric mucosa. This condition, known as follicular gastritis, is considered a form of chronic gastritis. HE.

Tumours

035A

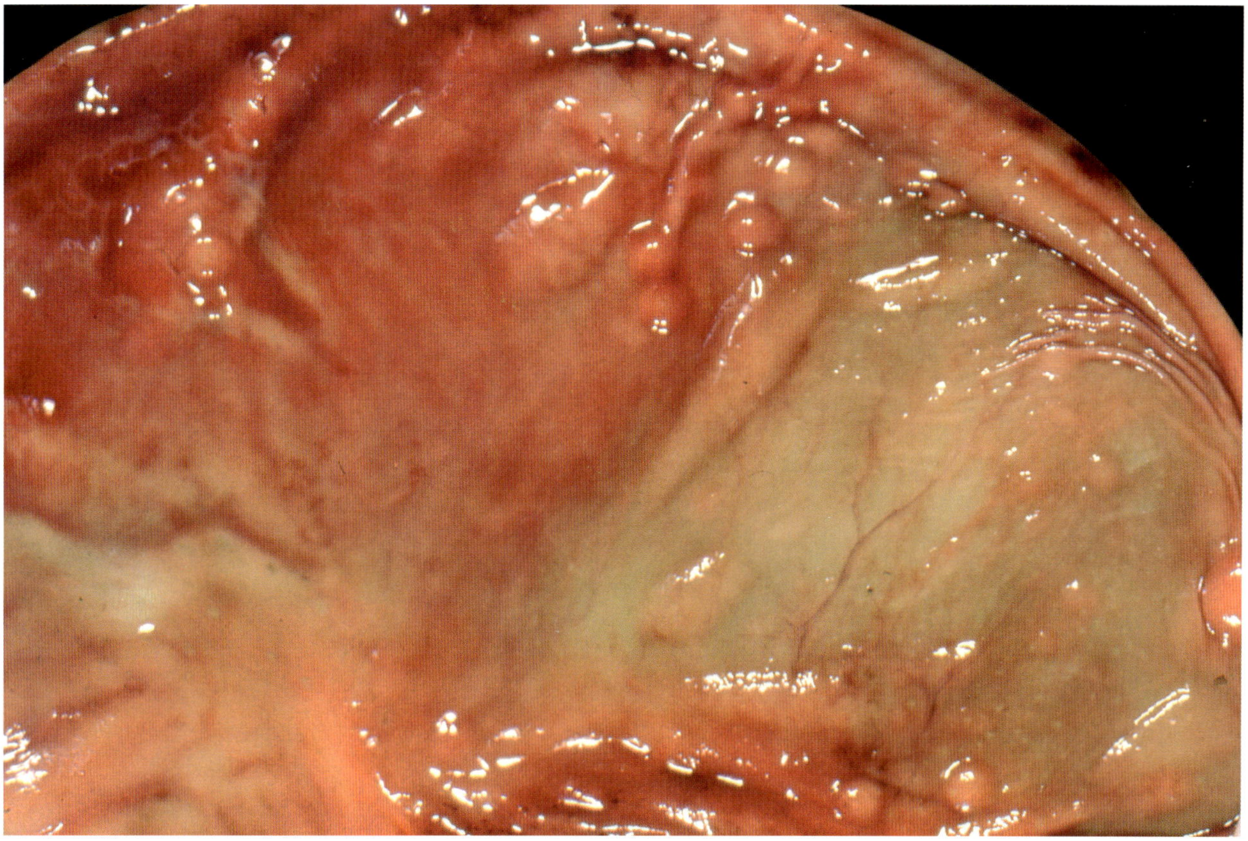

035A Intramural lymphoma.
Raised, multifocal nodules of variable size on the gastric mucosa. Fattening pig.

035B Intramural lymphoma.
Proliferation of lymphoid cells infiltrating the gastric wall and obliterating the structure of the organ. HE.

035B

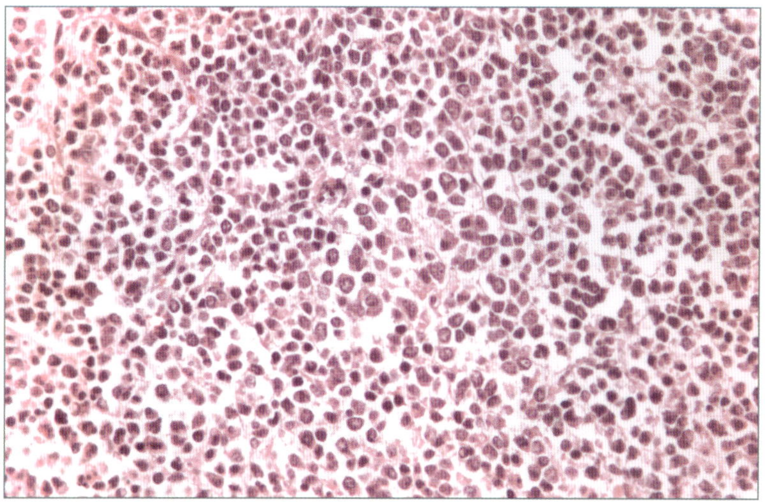

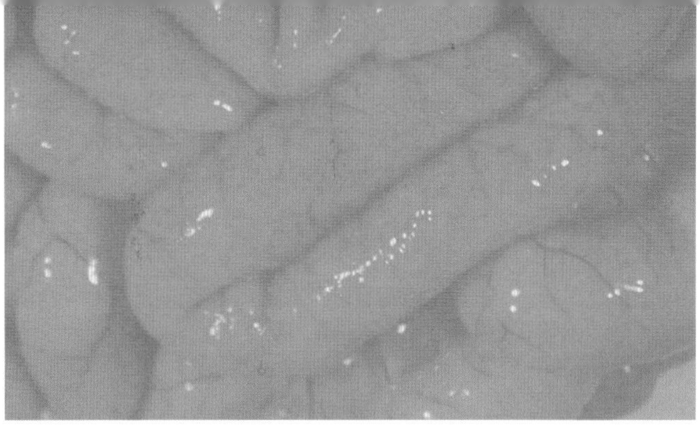

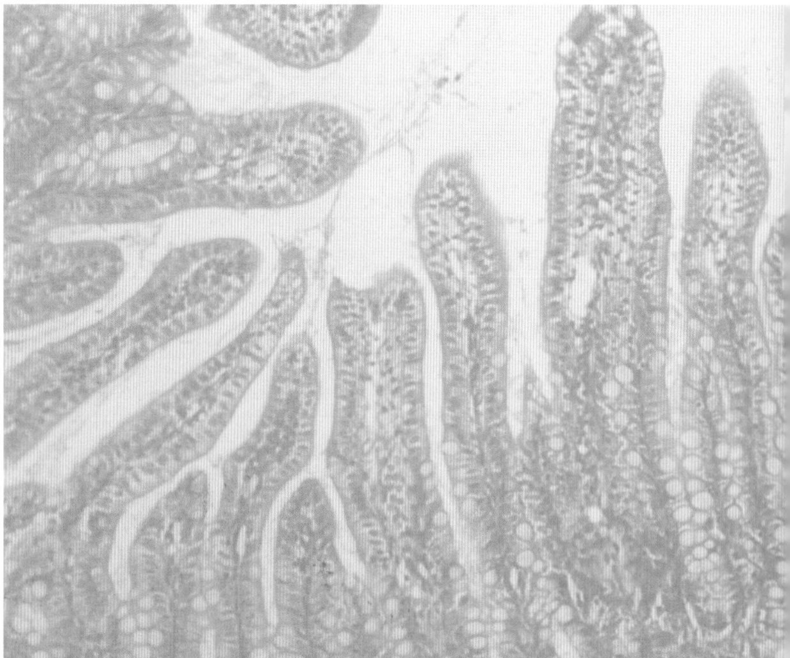

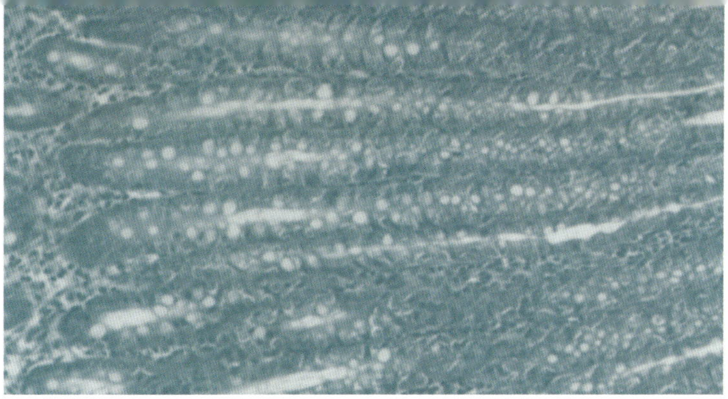

Intestine

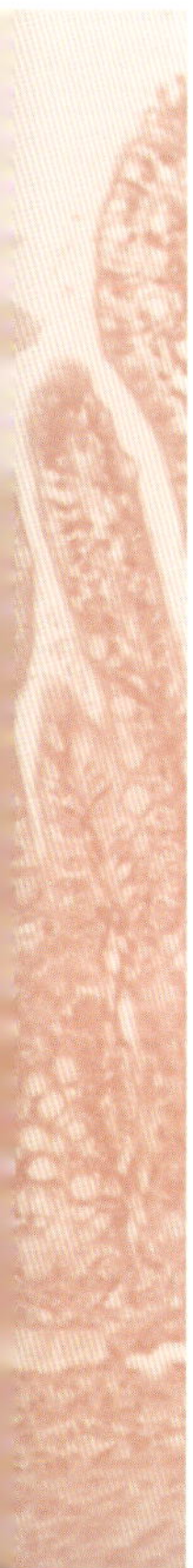

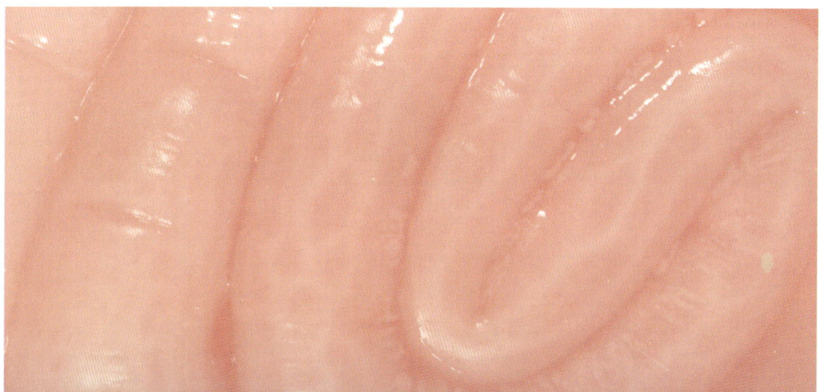

Postmortem changes

036

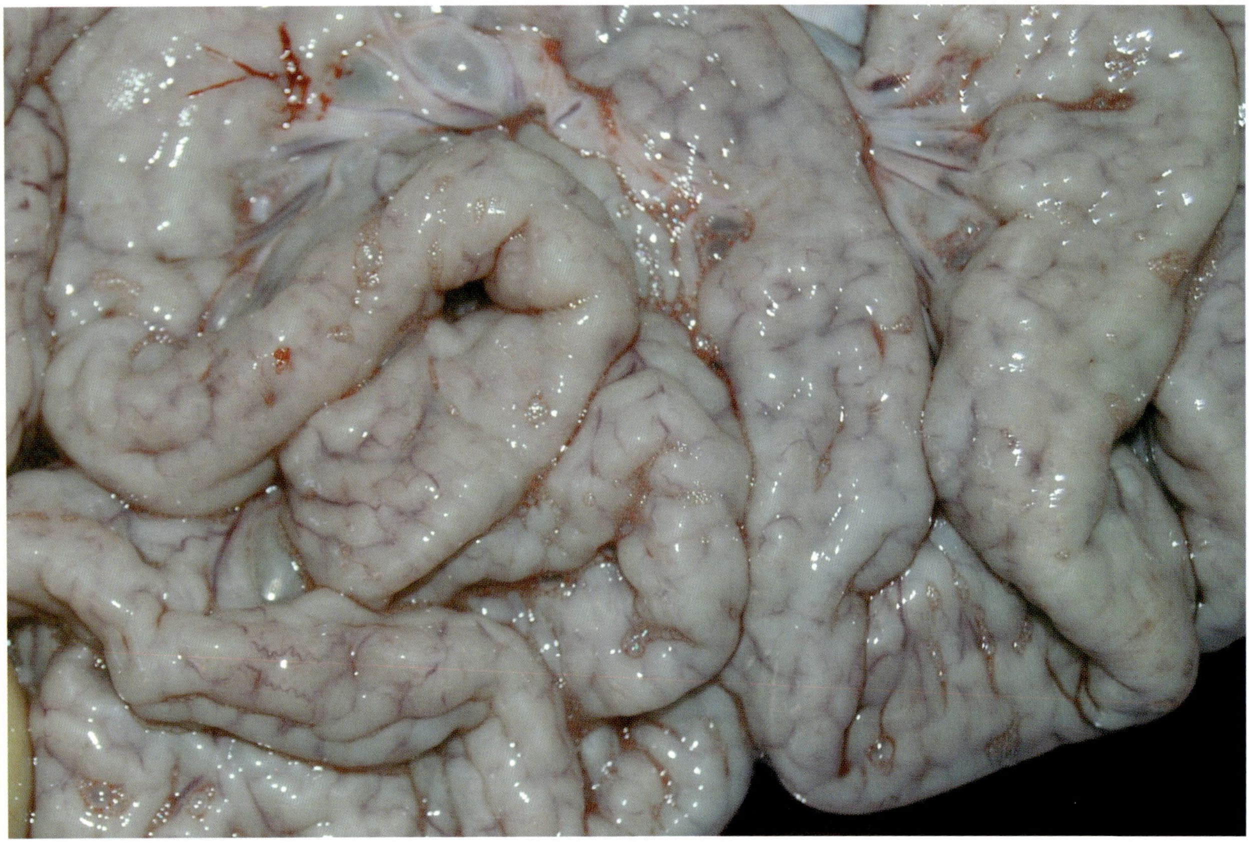

036 Terminal contraction.
Turgid loops of the small intestine appear reticulated due to the presence of marked folds in the mucosa.

037

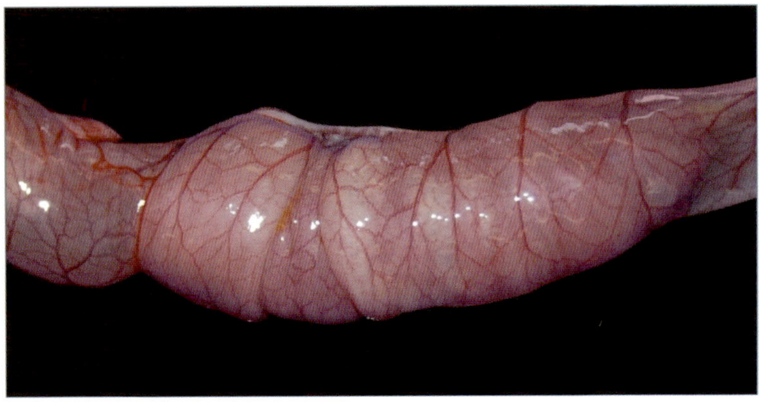

Intussusception and the contraction of intestinal segments are manifestations of irregular peristalsis immediately following the death of the animal. Terminal contraction is not caused by chronic inflammation and the folds disappear if stretched. False intussusception is recognised by the relative absence of circulatory disturbances.

037 Agonal intussusception.
Portion of the small intestine which is thickened due to the introduction into its lumen of an adjacent segment.

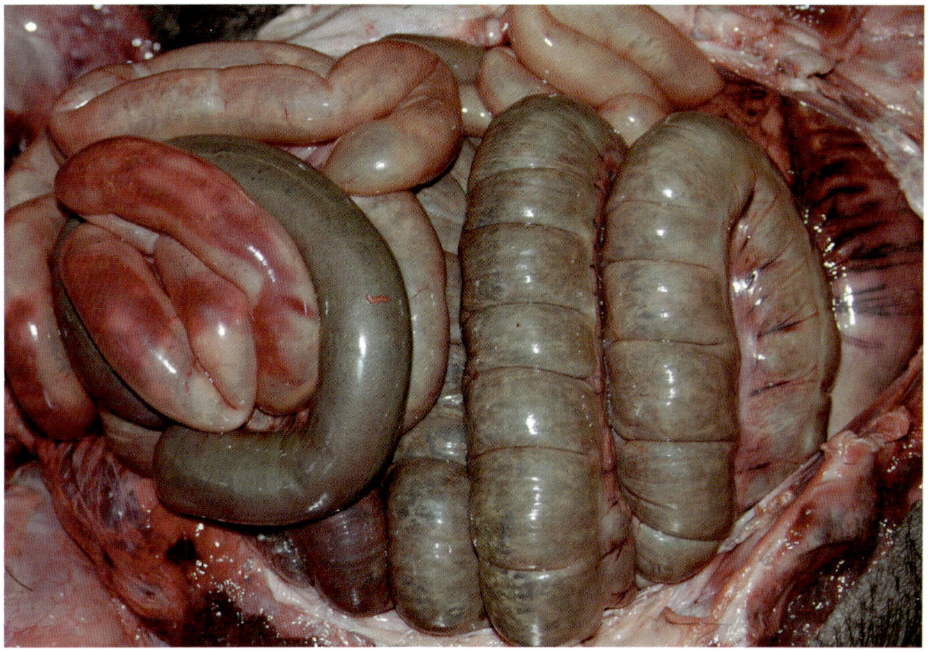

038

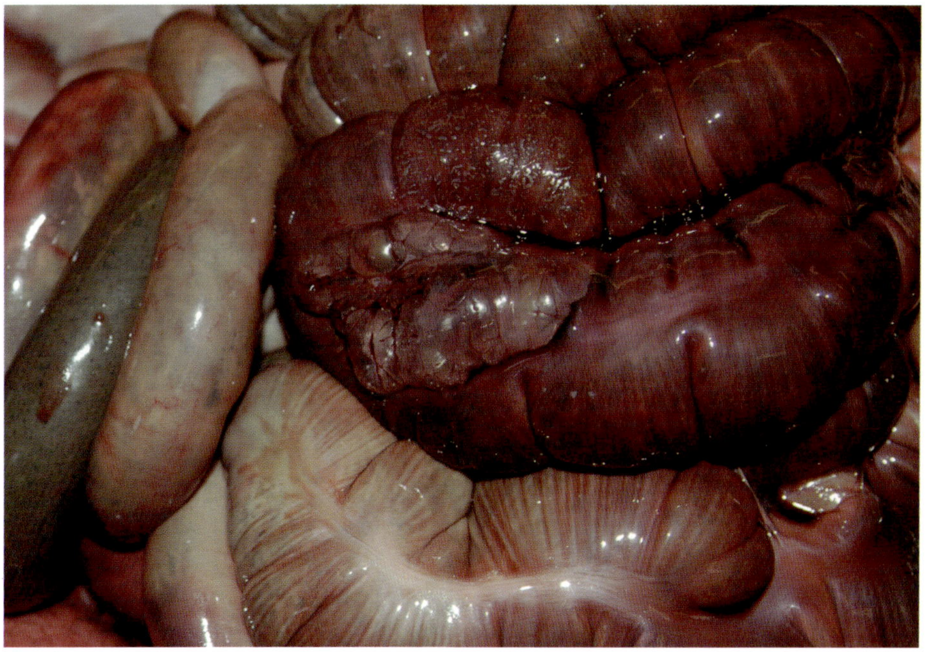

039

038 Postmortem bloating.
Late-stage, generalised insufflation of the intestine with discolouration, caused by gases produced by the action of bacteria on the intestinal contents.

039 Postmortem emphysema.
Formation of gas bubbles under the serosa of the large intestine due to the action of saprophytic bacteria, coupled with bloating and haemoglobin imbibition.

040

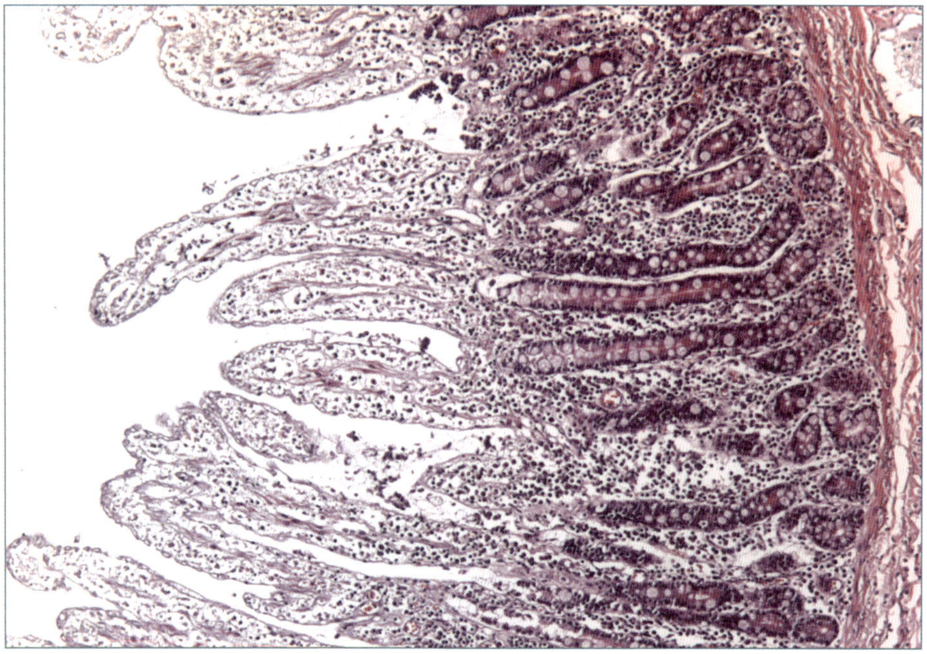

040
Autolysis.
The villi are devoid of epithelium, but the crypts are conserved. HE.

041

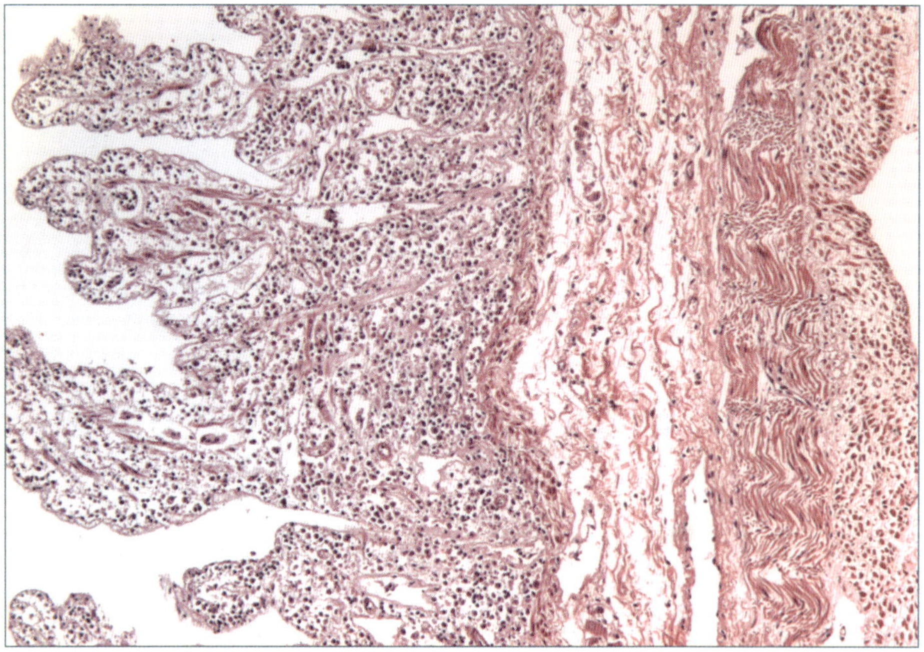

041
Autolysis.
Diffuse acidophilia of the wall of the small intestine with disorganisation of the mucosal layers and disappearance of the epithelium, villi, and crypts. HE.

The processes of autolysis and putrefaction occur rapidly in the intestine.
The loss of structural integrity limits or precludes interpretation of histological lesions.

Positional changes

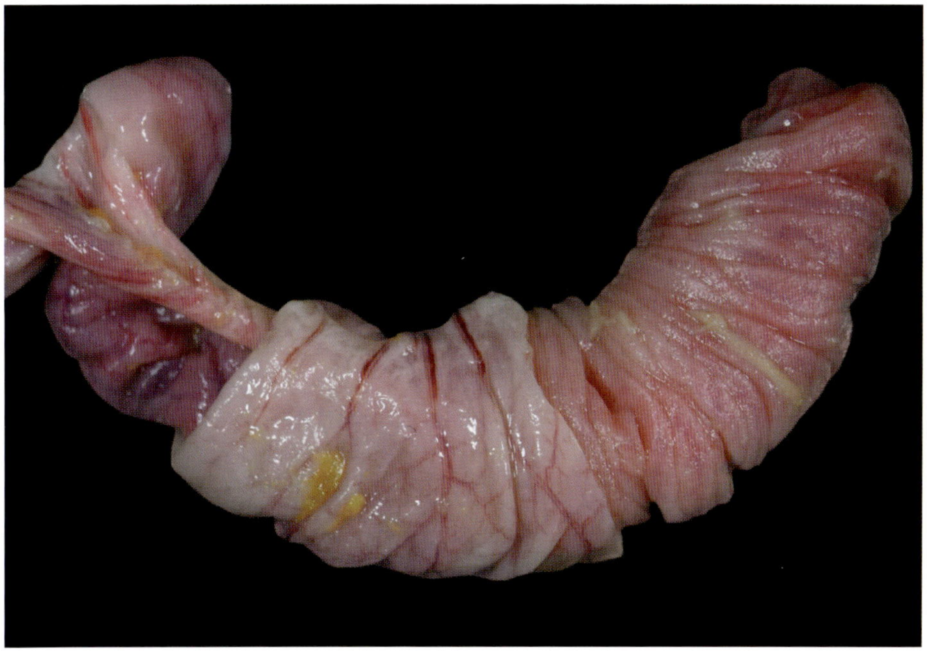

042

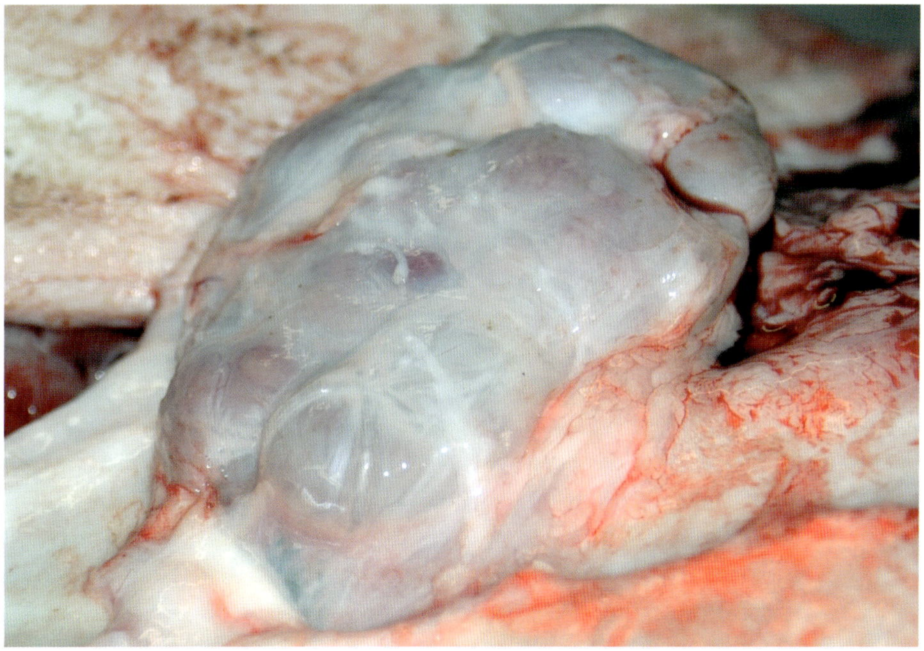

043

042 Enteric intussusception.
The affected segment has a turgid appearance due to the entry of one loop of the small intestine into the adjacent loop. The increase in colouration depends on the degree of vascular compromise.

043 External hernia.
Intestinal loops displaced outside the abdominal cavity, covered by the peritoneum.

Alterations of the lumen

044

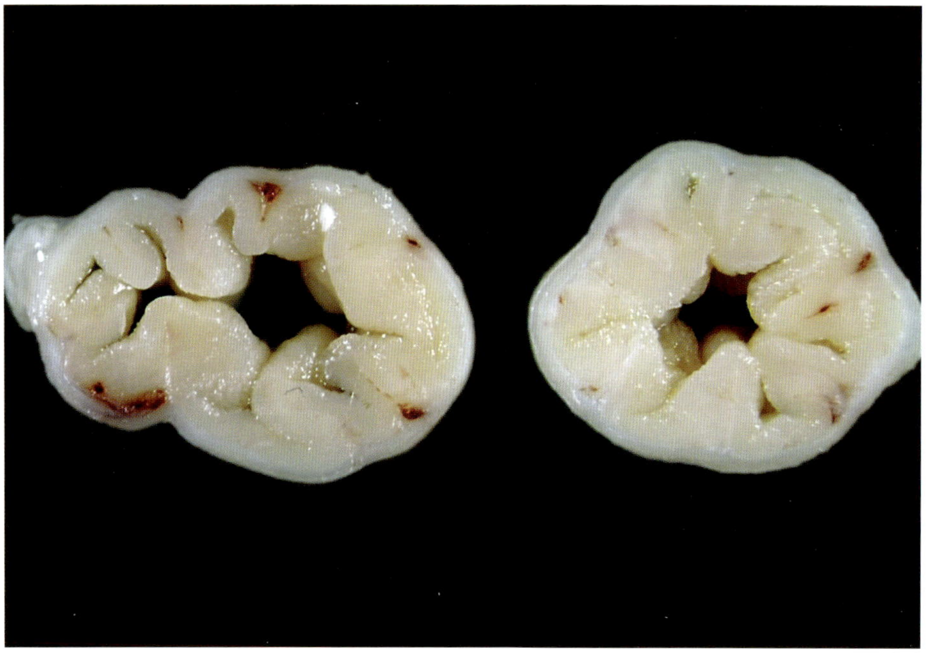

045

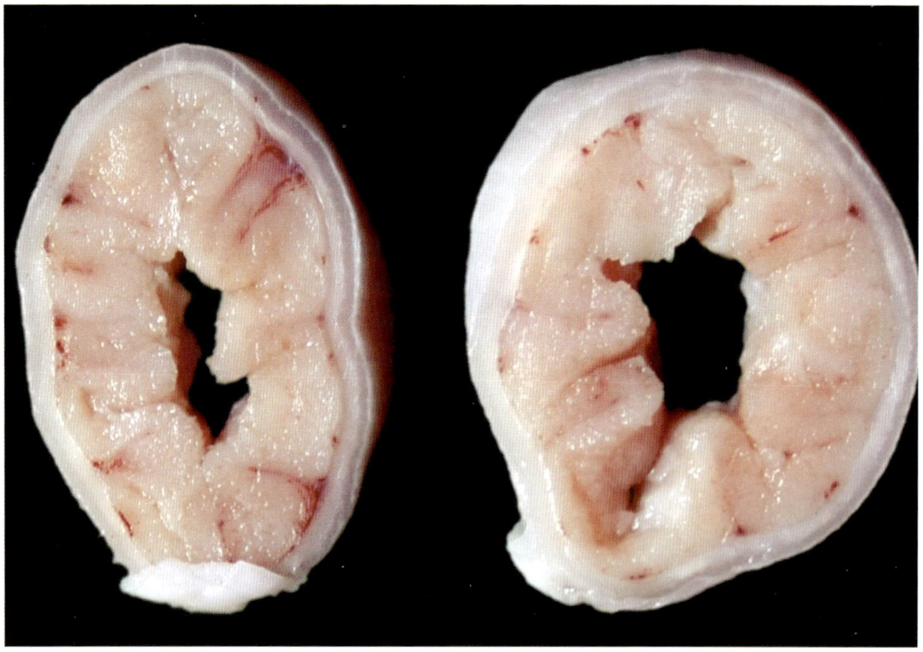

044 Stenosis.
Narrowing of the lumen of the small intestine due to mucosal thickening in a case of chronic inflammation. Fixed sample.

045 Stenosis.
Narrowing of the lumen of the small intestine due to proliferative thickening of the small intestine. Fixed sample.

046

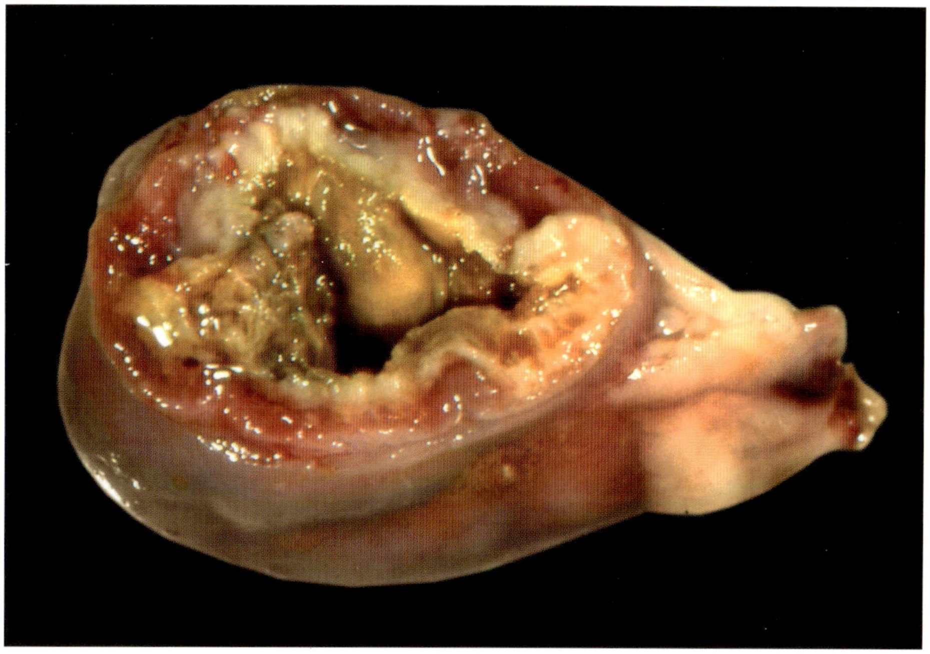

047

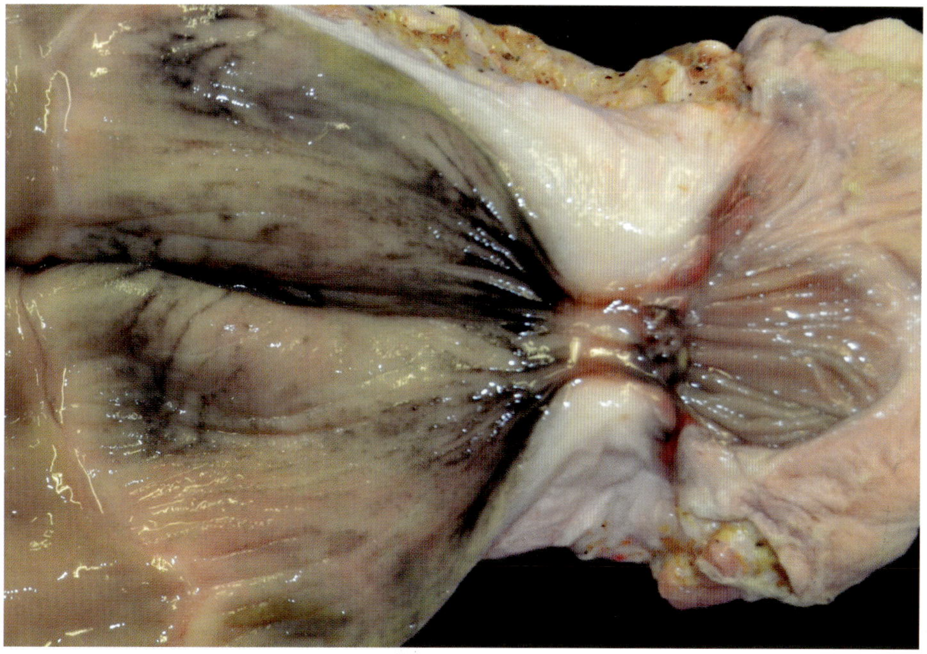

046 Stenosis.
Narrowing of the lumen of the small intestine due to the presence of a dense exudate on the proliferating mucosa.

047 Stenosis.
Narrowing of the lumen caused by a whitish annular band formed by scarring of the rectal wall.

048

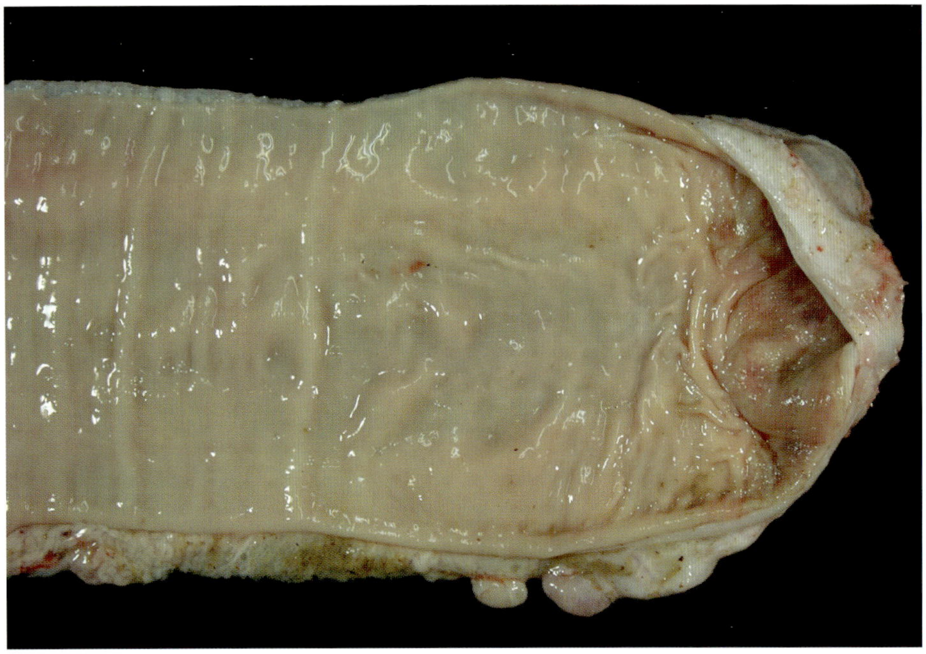

048 Occlusion.
Complete closure of the intestinal lumen as a result of rectal stenosis.

Stenosis is a sequela of lesions of the rectal mucosa, with the development of parietal fibrosis. This lesion is caused by enteric salmonellosis, amputation of rectal prolapse, mycotoxicosis, and other processes that compromise the local circulation via vasculitis and thrombosis.

049

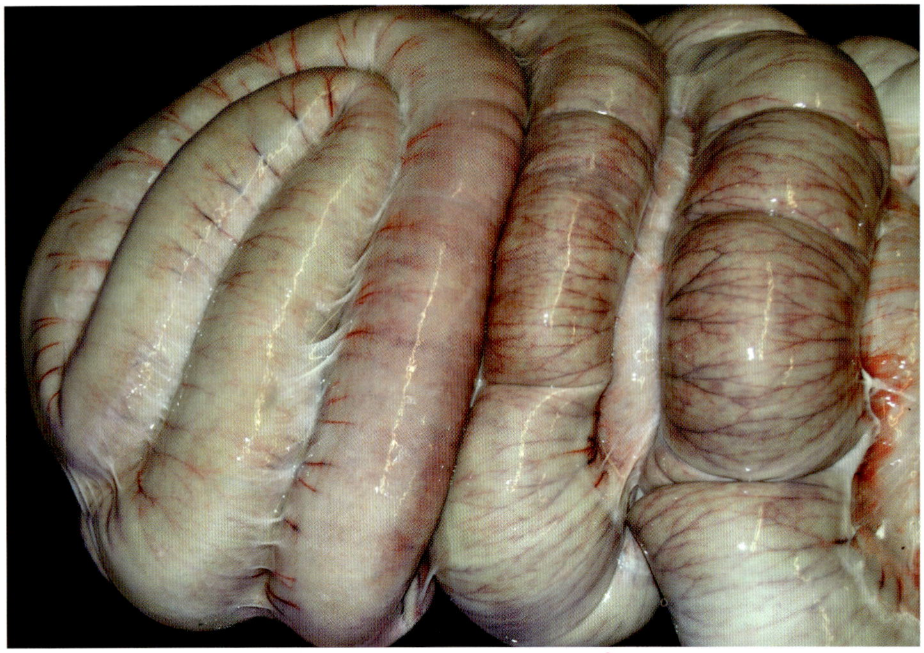

049 Dilation.
Expansion of the large intestine due to retention of its contents caused by rectal stenosis.

050 **Acquired megacolon.** Abnormal enlargement of the large intestine caused by dilation secondary to rectal stenosis.

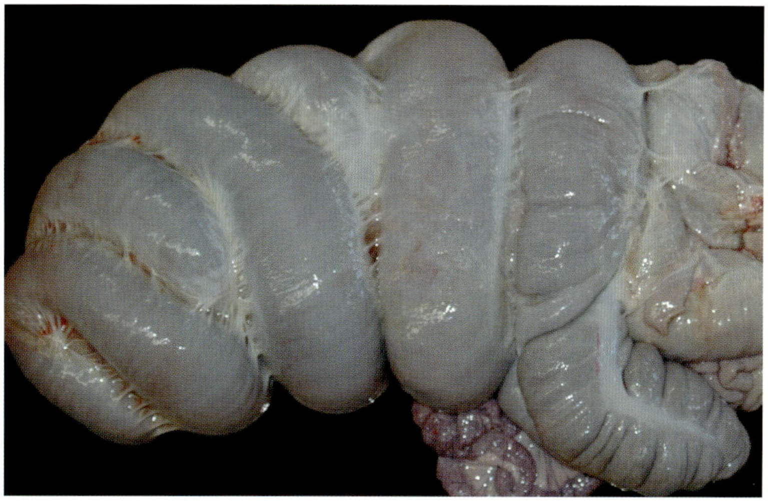

051A **Acquired megacolon.** Enlargement of the loops of the colon due to faecal accumulation secondary to rectal stenosis. Serosa with wrinkled appearance due to the presence of fibrous growths.

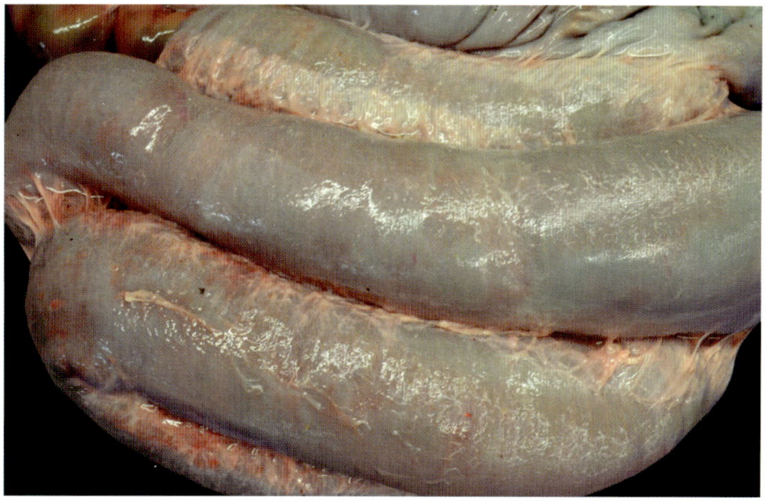

051B **Acquired megacolon.** The walls of the colon appear turgid and the mucosa is reddened.

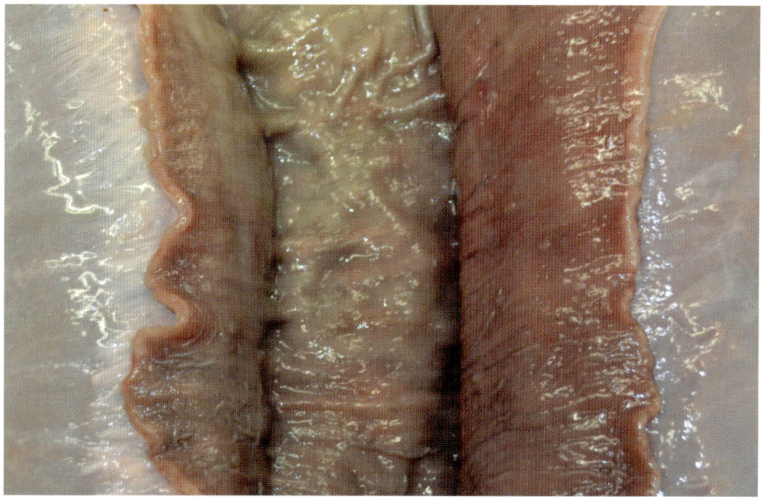

Acquired megacolon is usually a sequela of rectal stenosis and, in rare cases, can be caused by atonia.

Changes in content

052

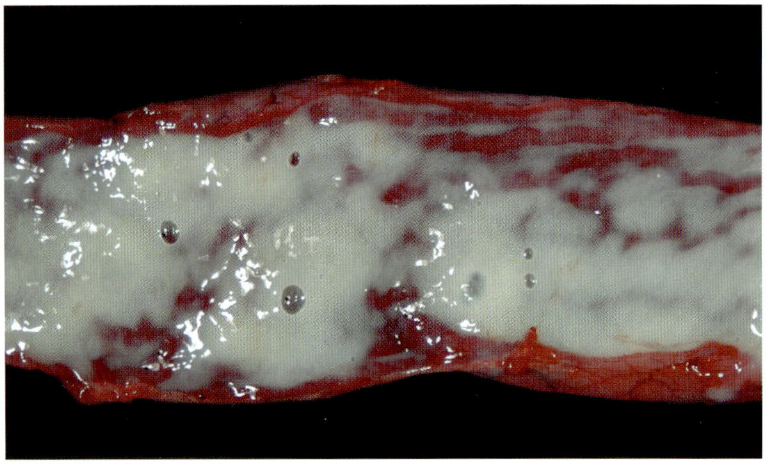

052 Content alterations.
Pasty, turbid, adherent deposits on the reddened mucosa of the small intestine in a case of acute inflammation.

053

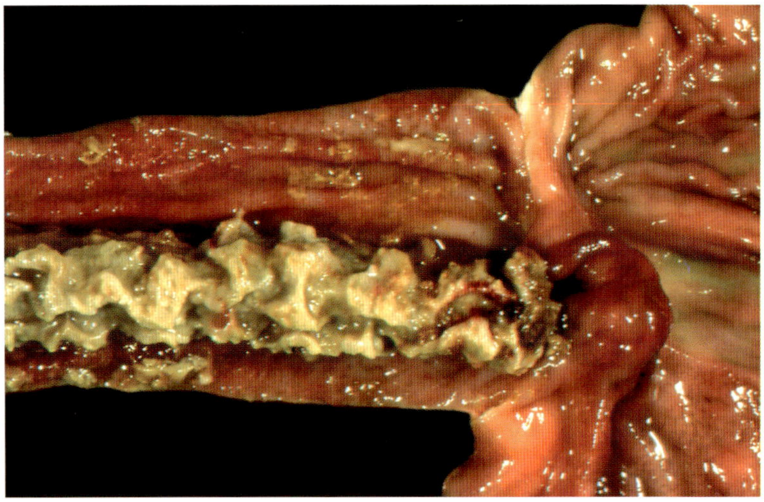

053 Abnormal contents.
Compact and anfractuous pseudomembranous exudate of the distal portion of the ileum that has been moulded by intestinal peristalsis.

Emphysema

054

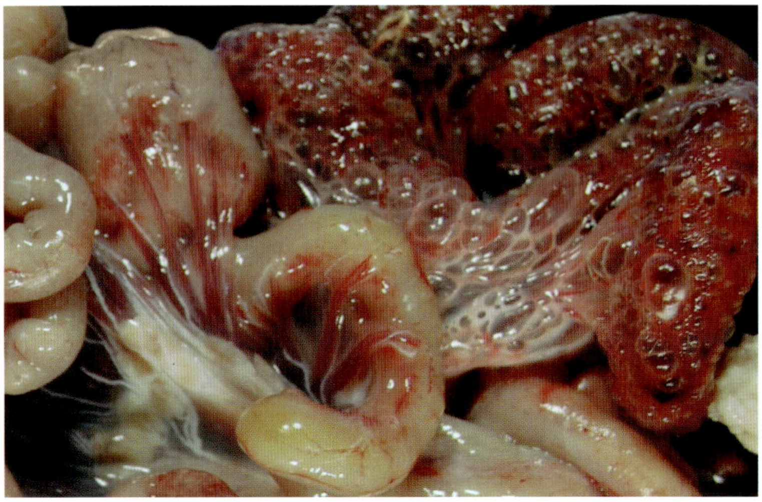

054 Emphysema.
A case of necrotic enteritis: the loops of the small intestine have an irregular surface due to the presence of bubbles in the intestinal wall and the mesentery. Suckling pig.

> In addition to the intestinal emphysema observed in enteritis, caused by the action of anaerobic bacteria, idiopathic emphysema is a sporadic finding of uncertain aetiology, with features of foreign body reaction.

Circulatory disorders

055 Oedema.

Abnormal separation of the mesocolon between two loops with tissue pallor in the affected area. Suckling pig. HE.

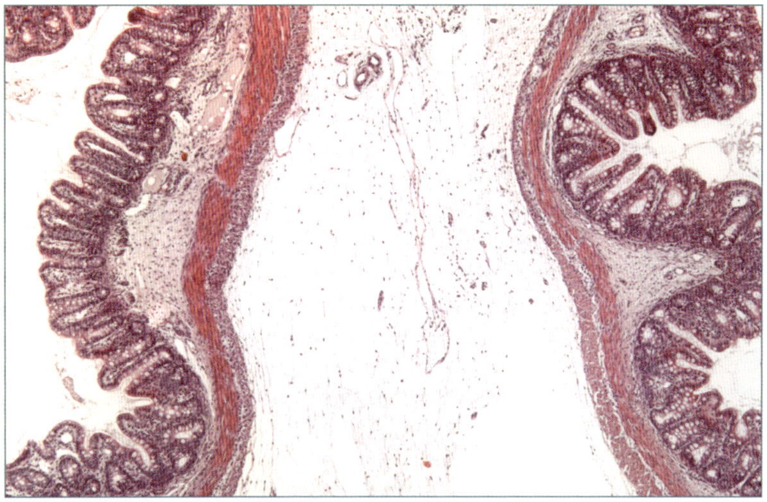

055

056 Oedema.

Expansion and tissue pallor in the submucosa of the colon. Suckling pig. HE.

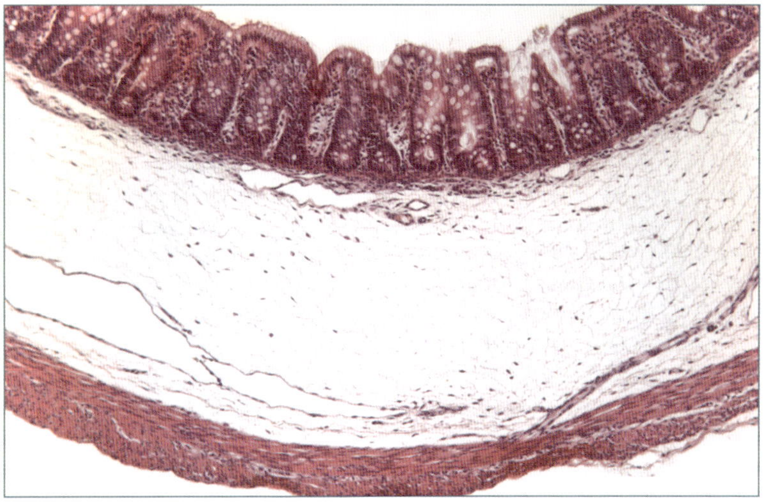

056

> Some forms of mesocolon oedema in suckling pigs may be due to the action of mycotoxins. Submucosal oedema can manifest throughout the entire intestine.

057 Oedema.

Gelatinous expansion caused by the accumulation of fluid between the loops of the colon in two suckling pigs.

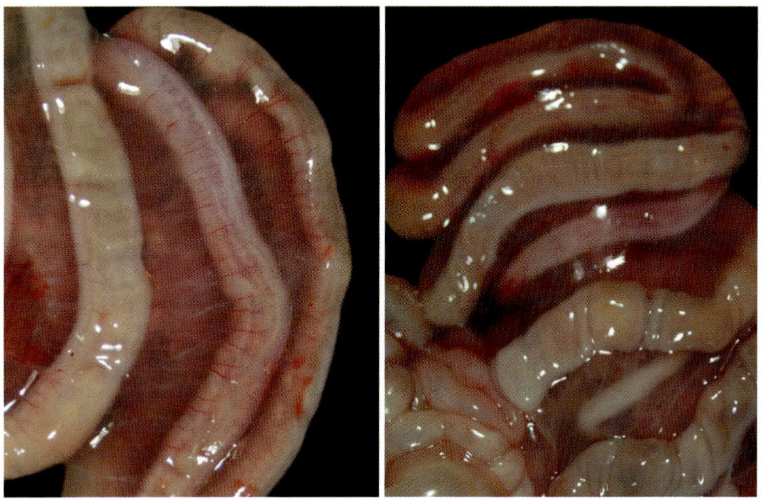

057

058A

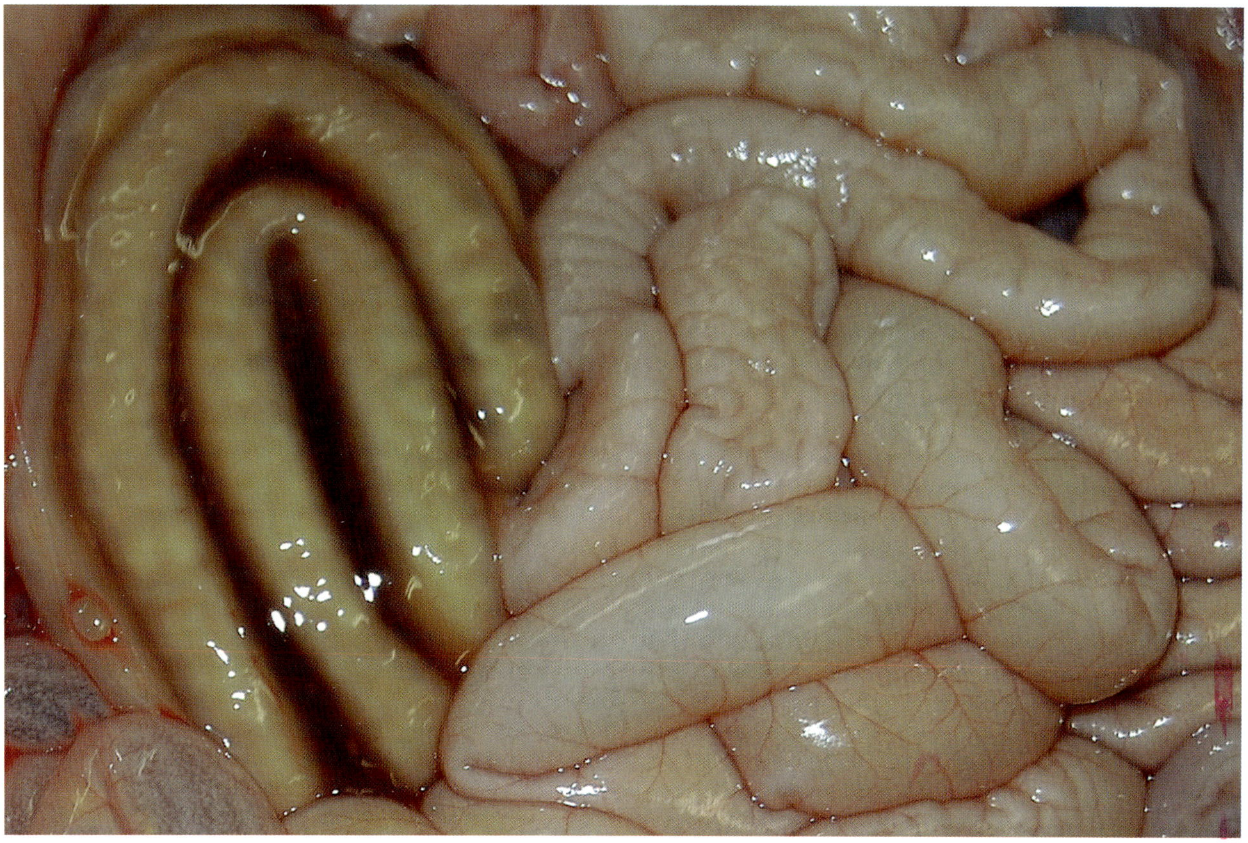

058A Oedema.
Gelatinous expansion of the mesocolon. Suckling pig.

058B

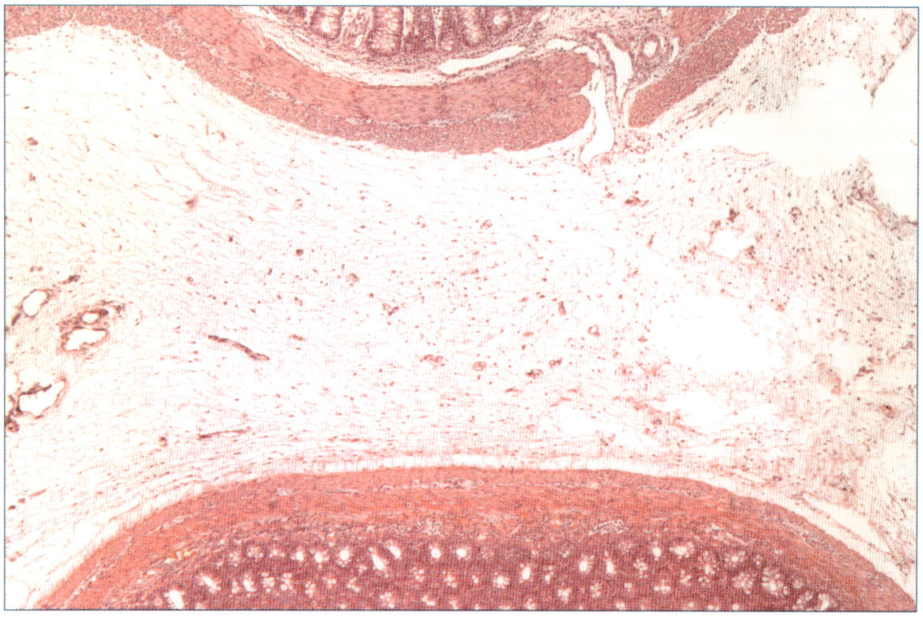

058B Oedema.
Expansion of tissue components between two loops of the colon caused by fluid accumulation. HE.

Mesocolon oedema, which is common in cases of *Clostridium difficile* infection in piglets, is not considered a pathognomonic indicator.

059A

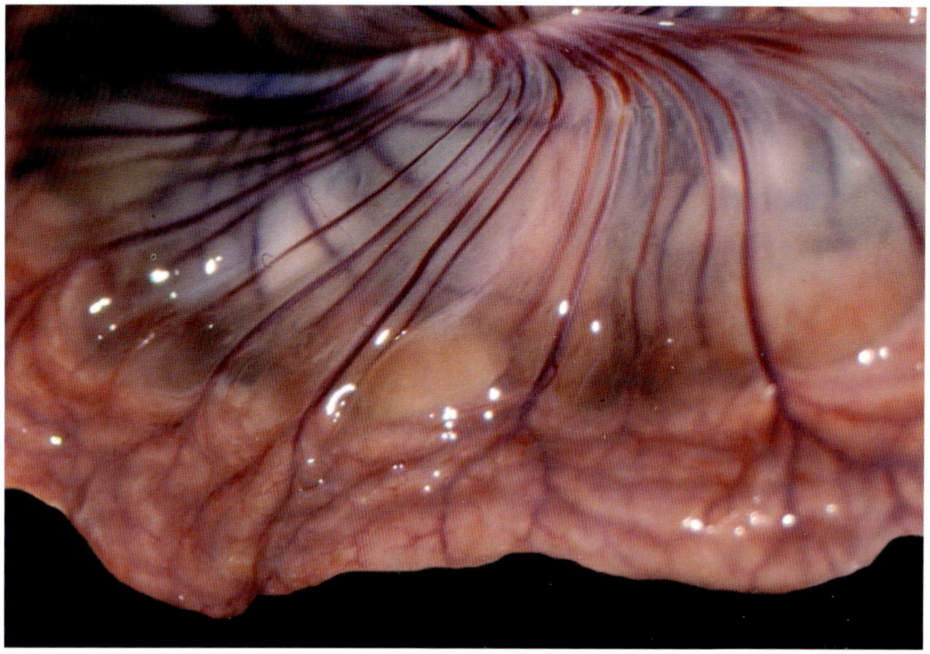

059B

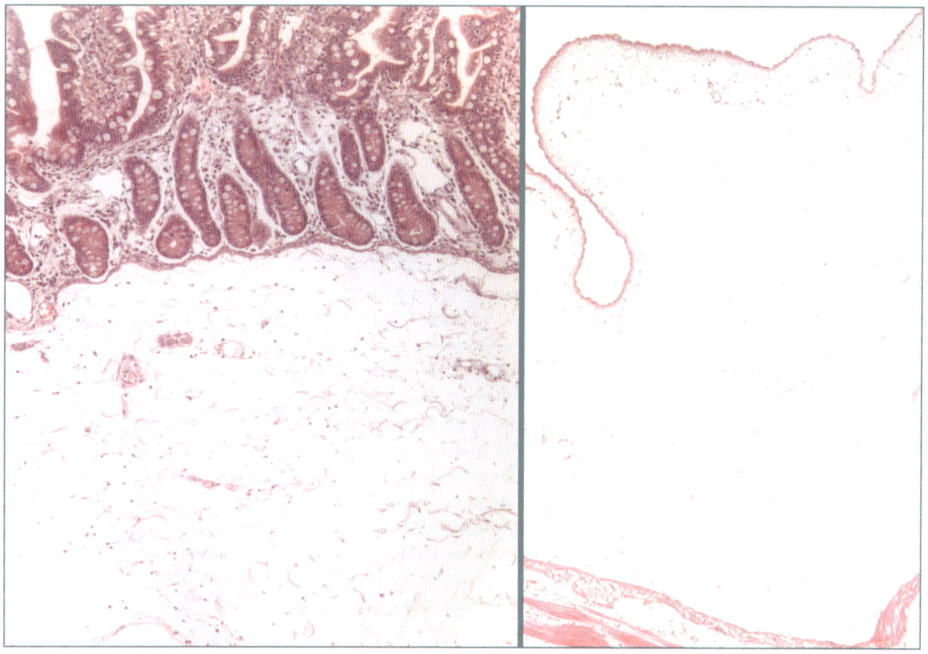

059A Oedema.
Gelatinous infiltration, more pronounced in the mesenteric insertion of the small intestine. Weaner pig.

059B Oedema.
Paleness of the submucosa due to expansion of the extracellular matrix (left). Separation of the serosa due to submesothelial accumulation of fluid (right). HE.

060

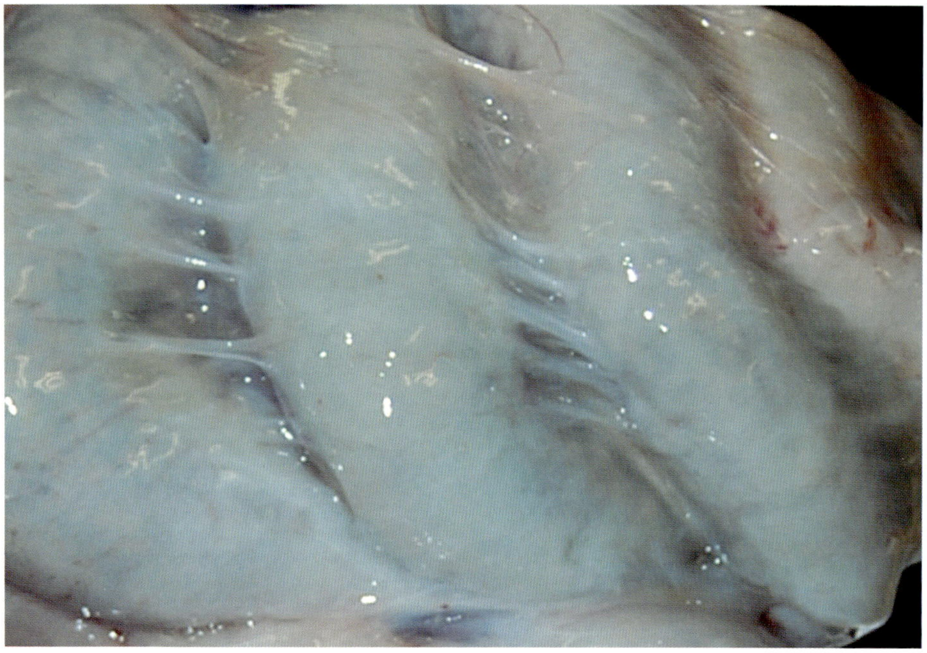

061

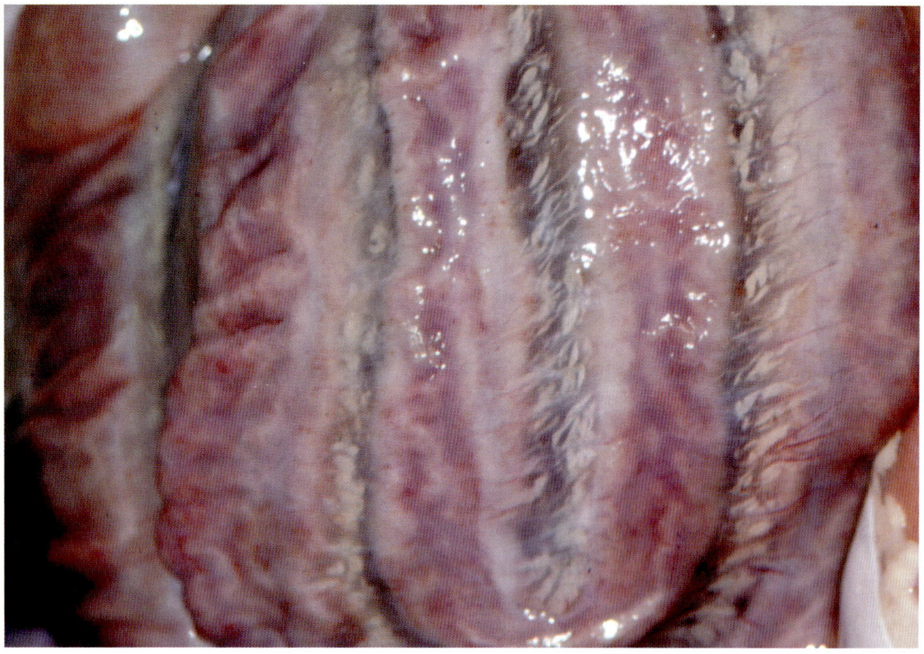

060 Oedema.
Expansion of the space between loops of the colon in a case of typhlocolitis. Weaner pig.

061 Oedema.
Loops of the colon separated by gelatinous bands. Weaner pig.

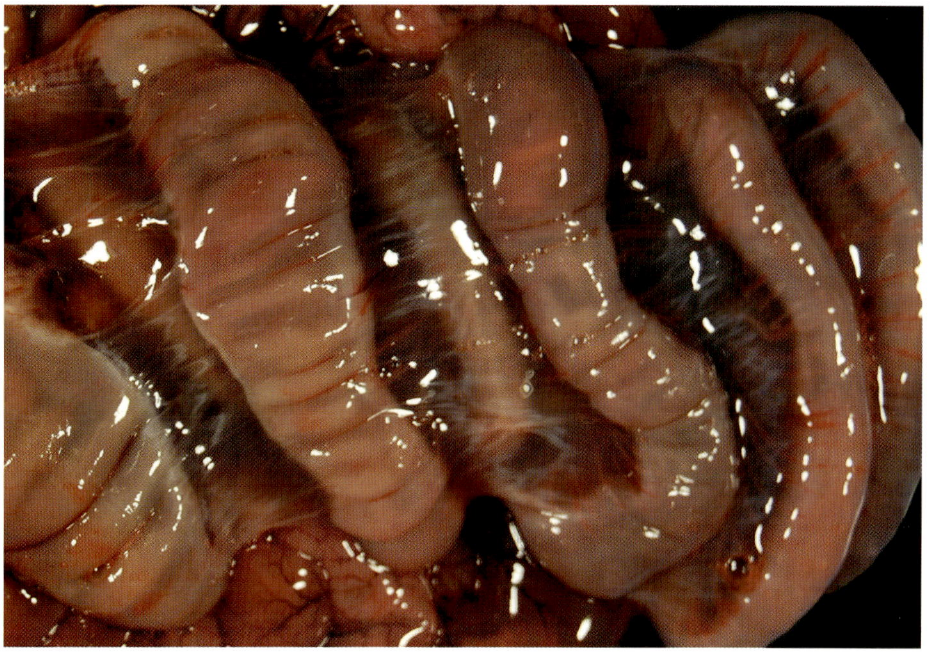

062A

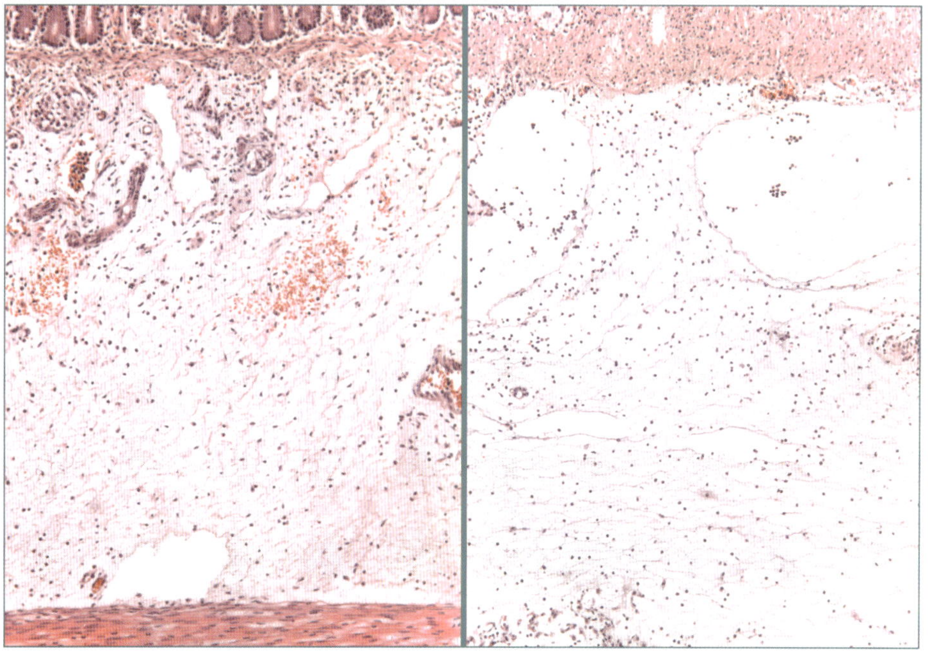

062B

062A Oedema.
Dilated mesocolon with separation of the loops and gelatinous-looking serosa in a case of typhlocolitis. Weaner pig.

062B Oedema.
Submucosa with free erythrocytes and inflammatory cells scattered among the components of the expanded connective tissue (left). Enlargement of the subserosa due to fluid accumulation (right). HE.

063A

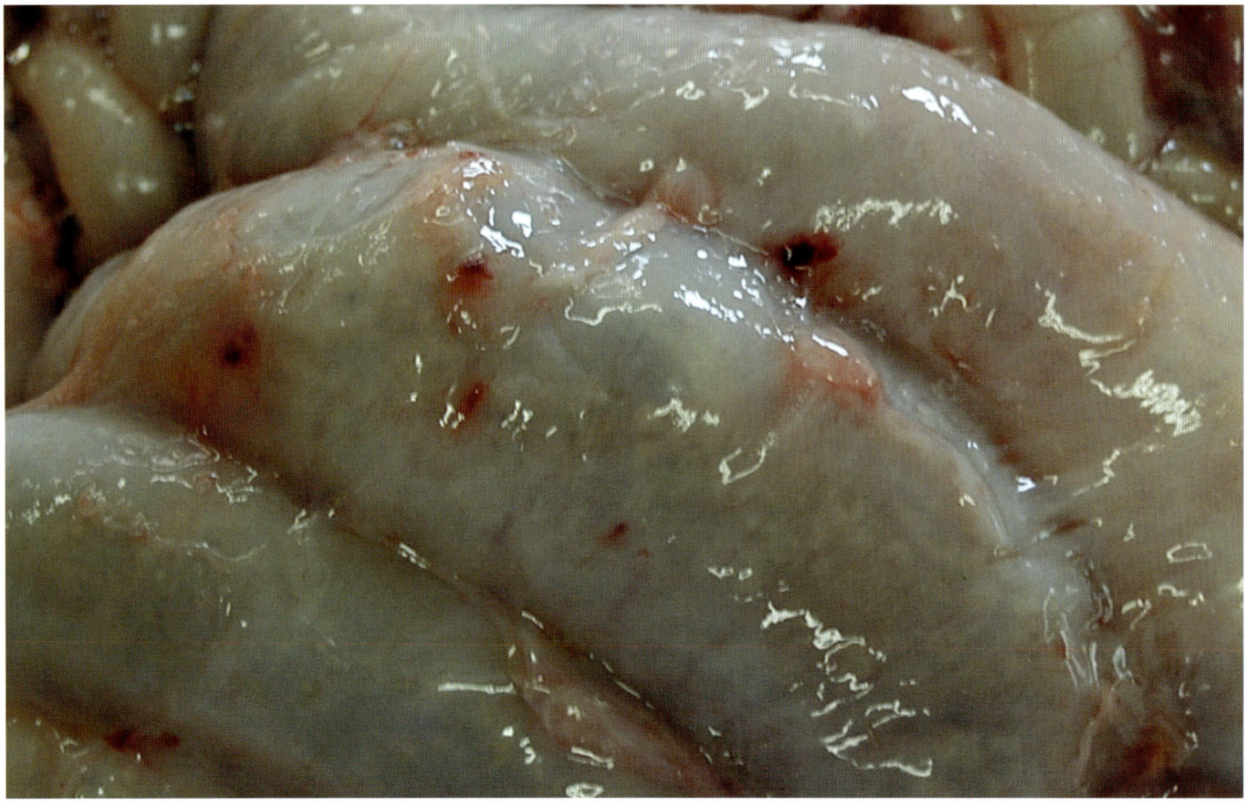

063A Oedema.
Colon with gelatinous-looking serosa and irregular surface in a case of typhlocolitis. Weaner pig.

063B

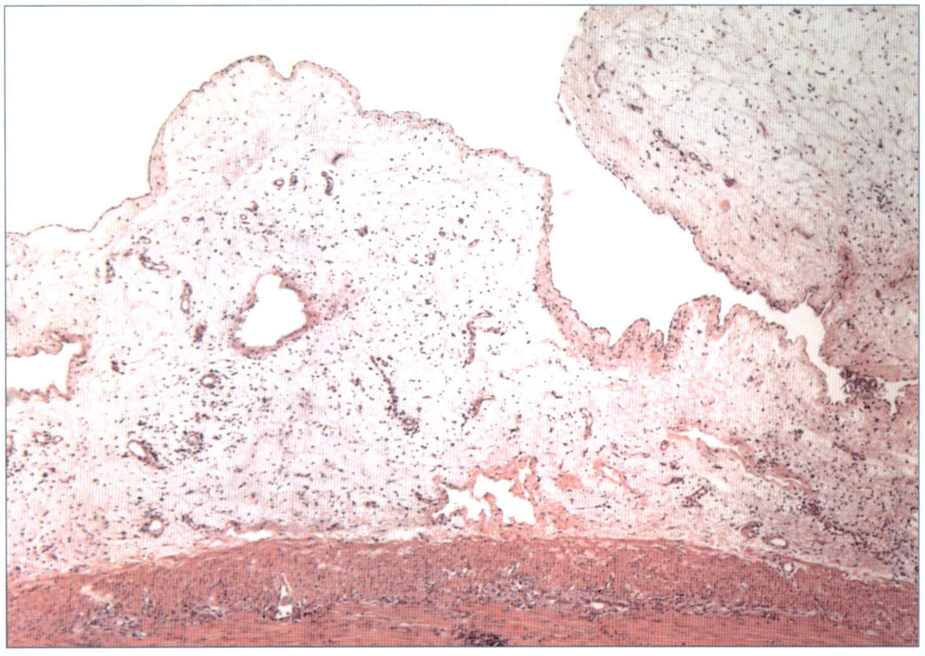

063B
Oedema.
Enlarged subserosa of irregular width due to the accumulation of fluid and the separation of tissue components. HE.

Mesocolon and mesenteric oedema can occur in oedema disease, salmonellosis, dysentery, spirochetosis, circovirosis, and trichuriasis, among other diseases. This lesion is also associated with hypoproteinaemia and circulatory disturbances.

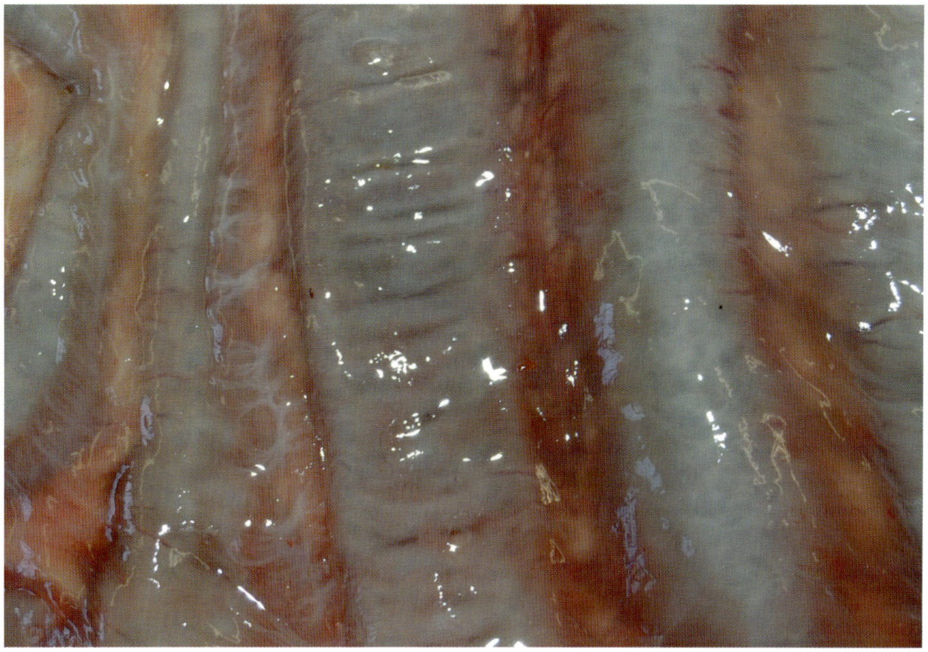

064

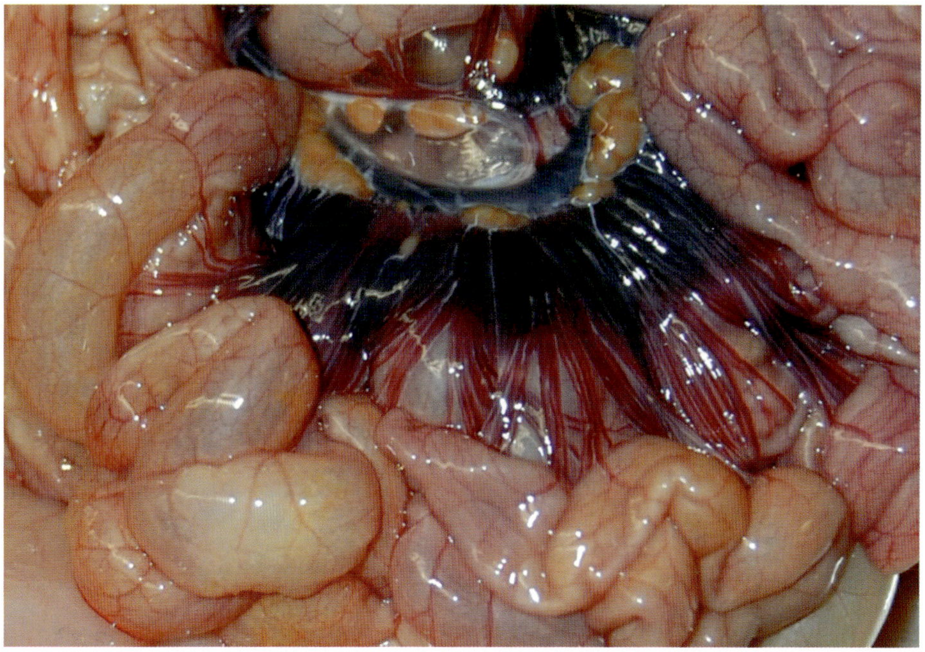

065

064 Oedema.
Enlarged and reddened gelatinous-looking mesocolon in a case of typhlocolitis. Fattening pig.

065 Hyperaemia.
Prominent, dilated mesenteric vessels. Suckling pig.

066

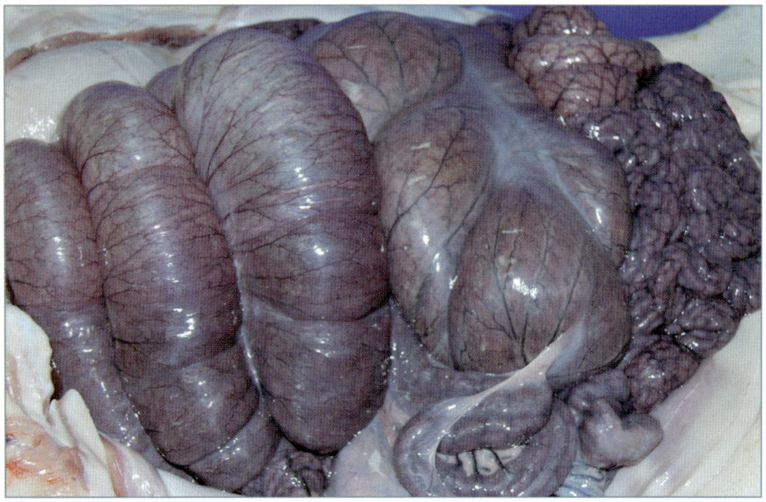

066 Hyperaemia.
Diffuse redness of the intestine in a case of acute inflammation. Weaner pig.

067A

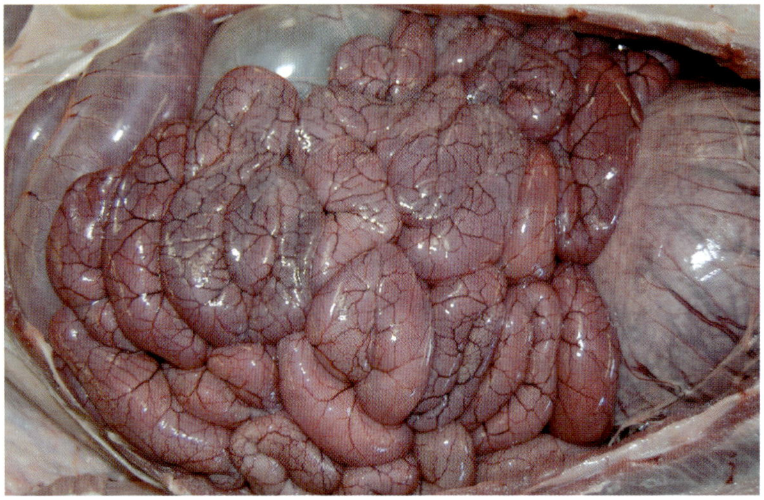

067A Hyperaemia.
Intestinal loops showing a diffuse increase in colour, with prominent vessels. Weaner pig.

067B

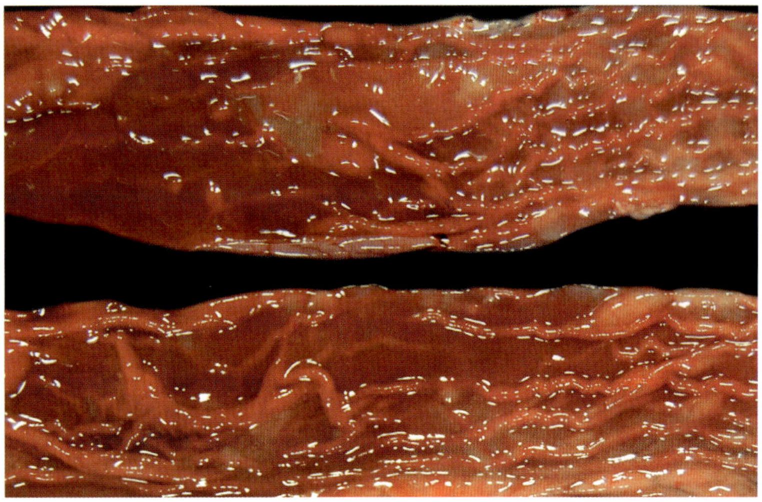

067B Hyperaemia.
Diffuse redness of the mucosa of the small intestine.

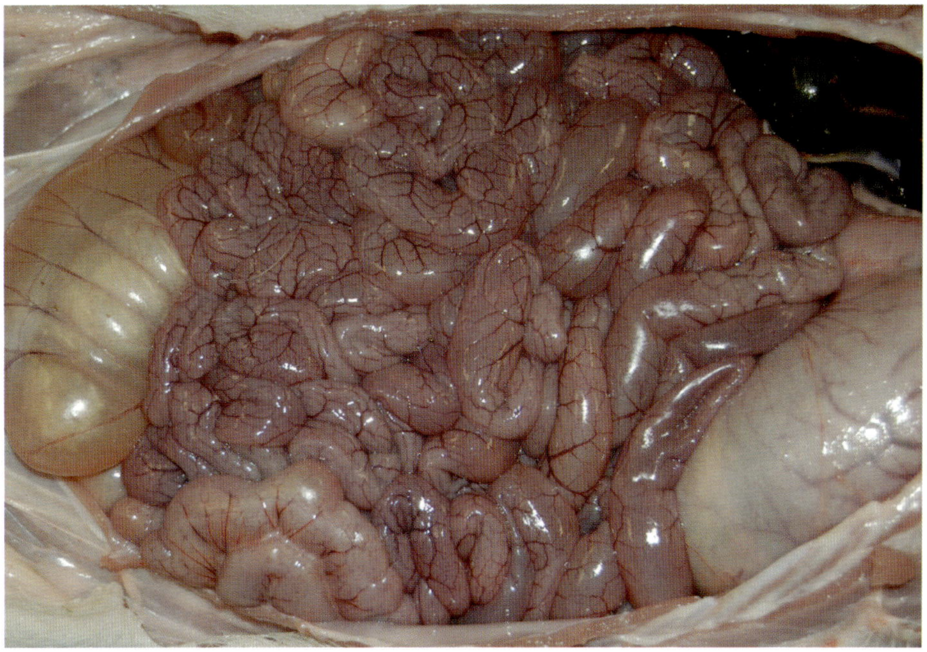

068A

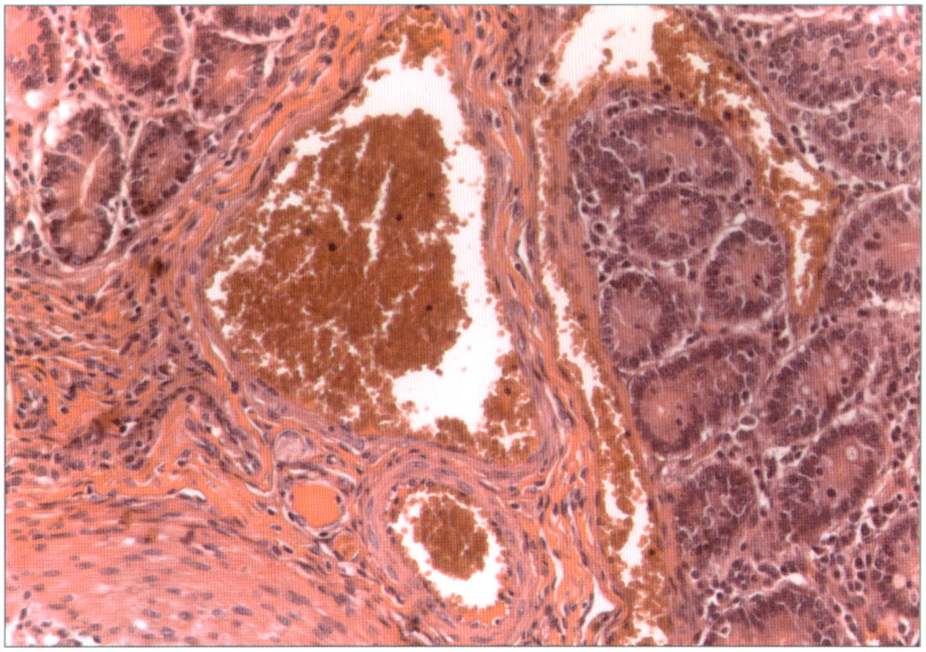

068B

068A **Hyperaemia.**
Increase in colour of the loops of the small intestine, with prominent blood vessels. Weaner pig.

068B **Hyperaemia.**
Dilated blood vessels of the lamina propria and submucosa containing abundant erythrocytes. HE.

069A

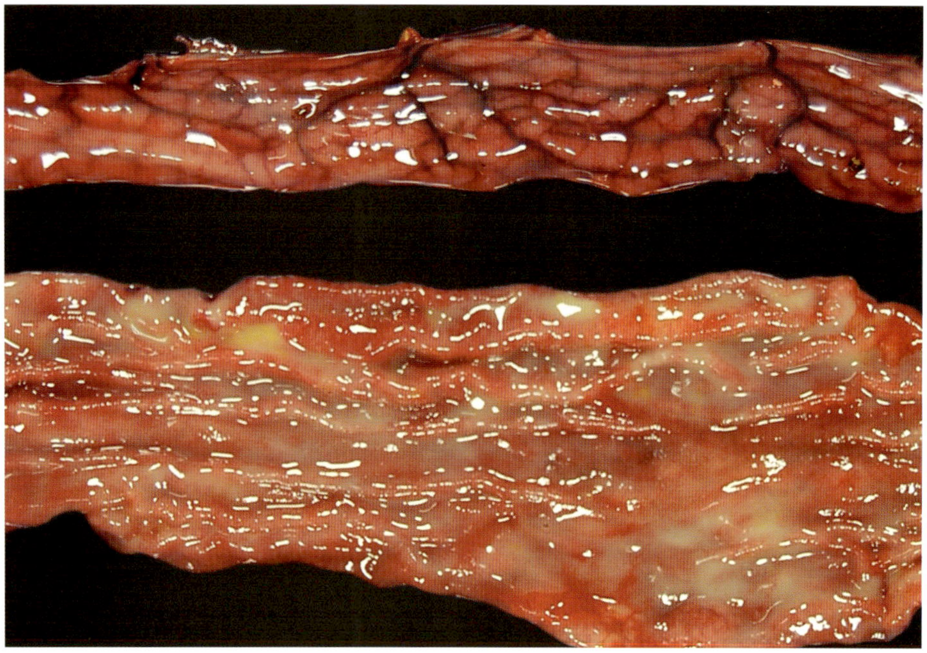

069B

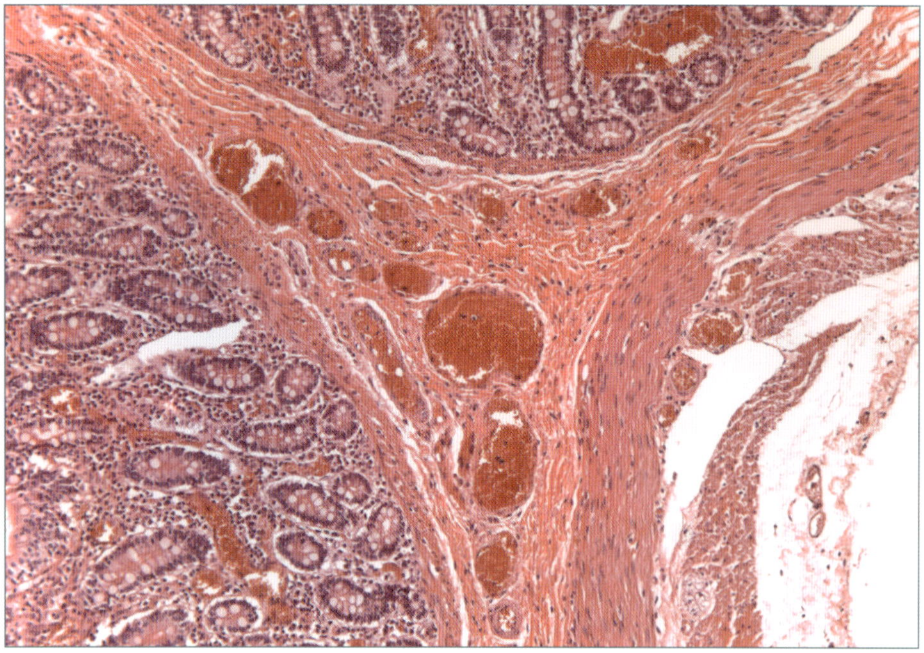

069A Hyperaemia.
Reddened serosa of the small intestine, with engorged blood vessels. Reddened mucosa with mucoid exudate.
Fattening pig.

069B Hyperaemia.
Dilated blood vessels of the lamina propria and submucosa containing abundant erythrocytes. HE.

070A Hyperaemia.
The vascular network of the small intestine is clearly visible through the mucosa.

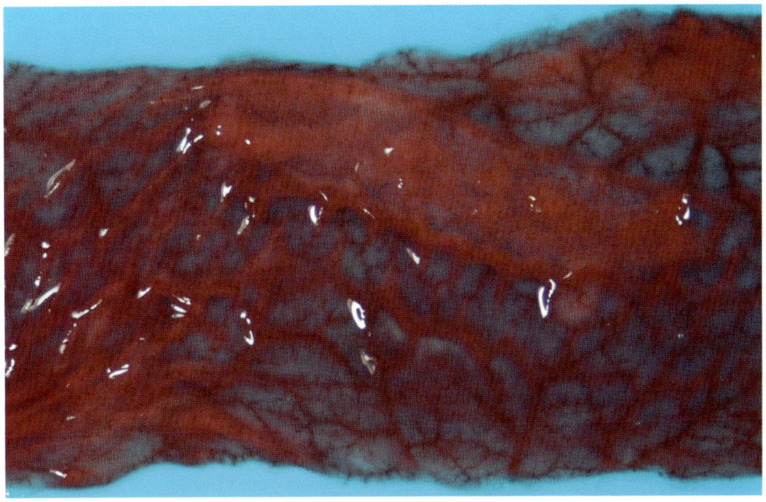
070A

070B Hyperaemia.
Dilated blood vessels of the submucosa containing abundant erythrocytes. HE.

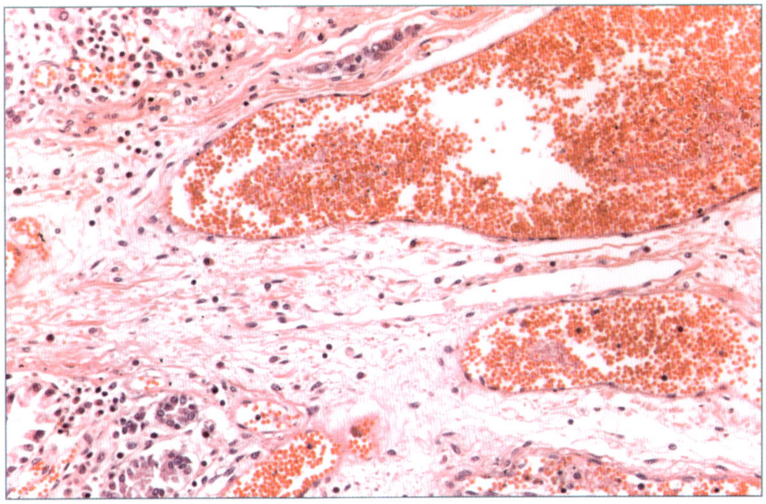
070B

071 Hyperaemia.
Diffuse reddening of the colonic mucosa in the acute phase of typhlocolitis. Fattening pig.

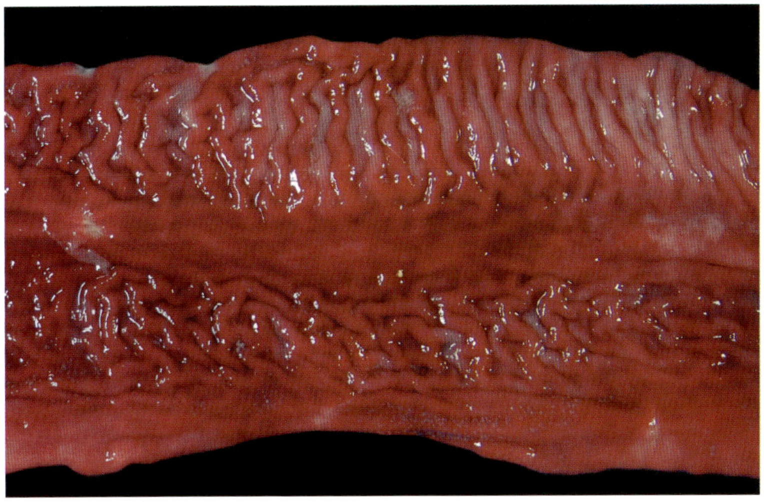
071

Pathological active hyperaemia occurs during the acute phase of intestinal inflammation. Passive hyperaemia is associated with heart failure, intestinal intussusception, and intestinal volvulus.

072

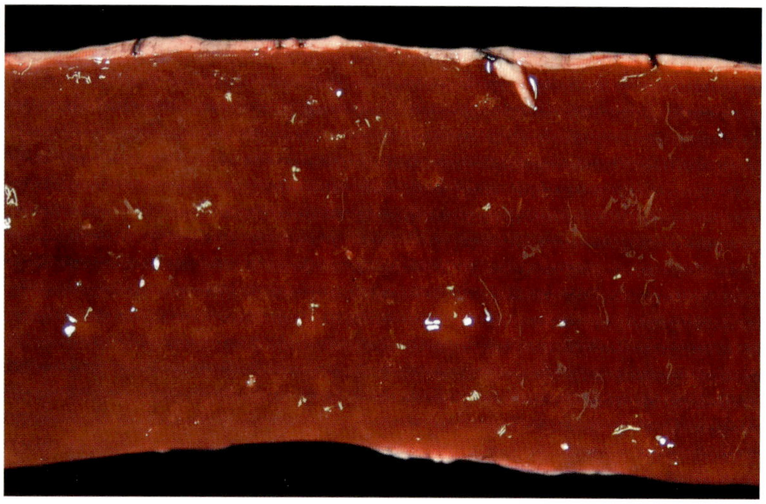

072 **Circulatory alterations.**
Intestinal mucosa showing diffuse redness. This sign can be associated with hyperaemia and/or haemorrhage.

073

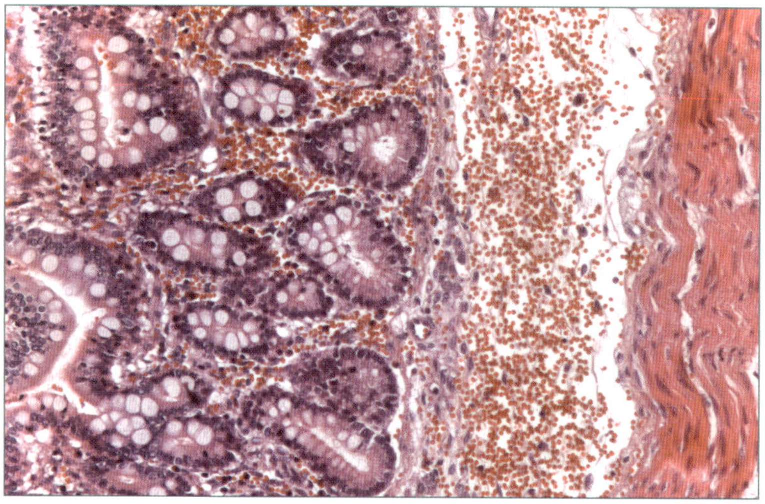

073 **Haemorrhage.**
Extravasation of erythrocytes in the lamina propria and submucosa of the small intestine. HE.

074

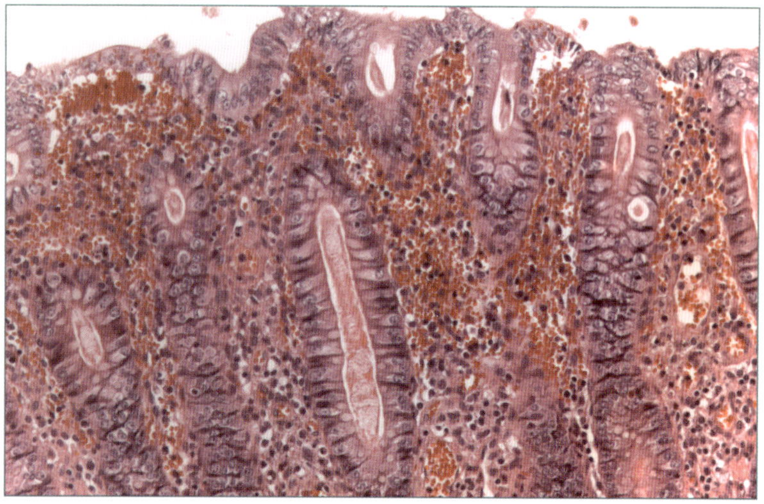

074 **Haemorrhage.**
Diffuse extravasation of erythrocytes in the lamina propria of the large intestine. HE.

075 Haemorrhage.
Dark red, diffusely dilated intestinal segments. Fattening pig.

Haemorrhage per rhexis can be caused by trauma or parasites. Haemorrhage per diapedesis occurs in cases of inflammation, septicaemia, swine fever, toxicosis, and infarction. In intestinal distension syndrome torsion is not considered necessary for diagnosis.

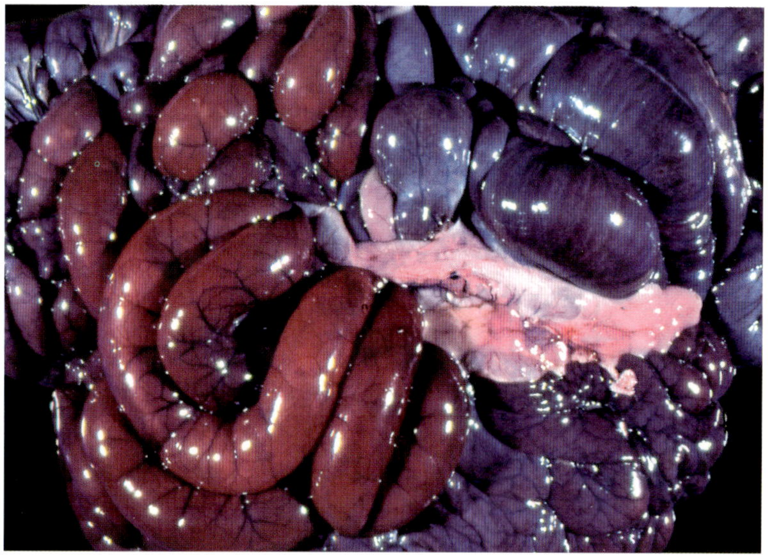
075

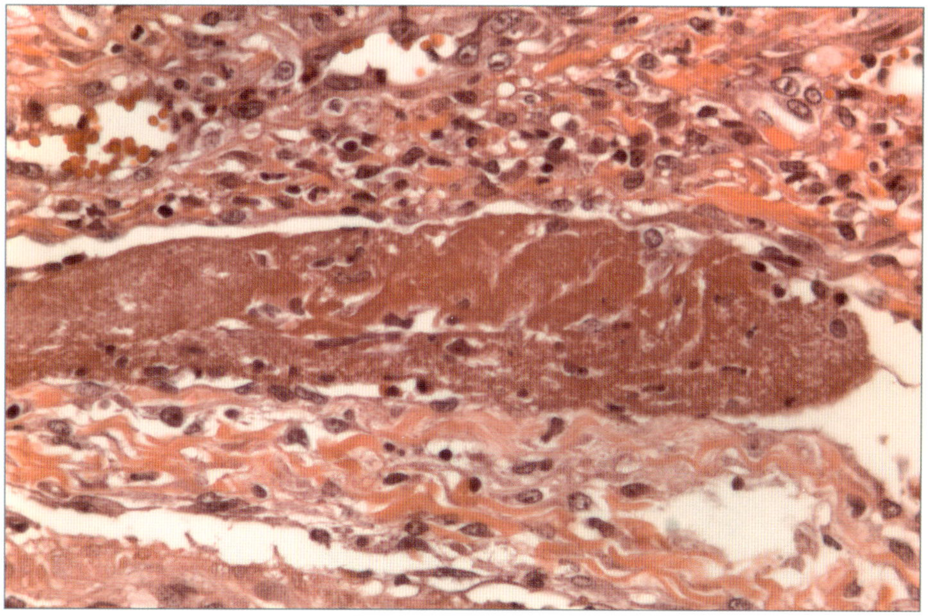
076

076 Thrombosis.
Coagulated mass occupying the lumen of a vessel in the intestinal submucosa in a case of typhlocolitis. HE.

077

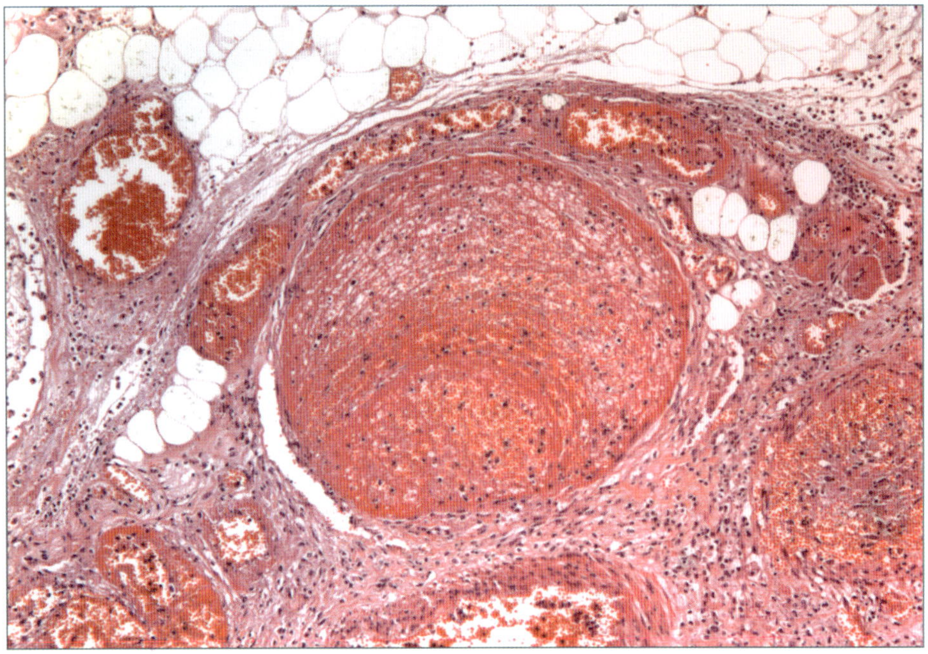

078

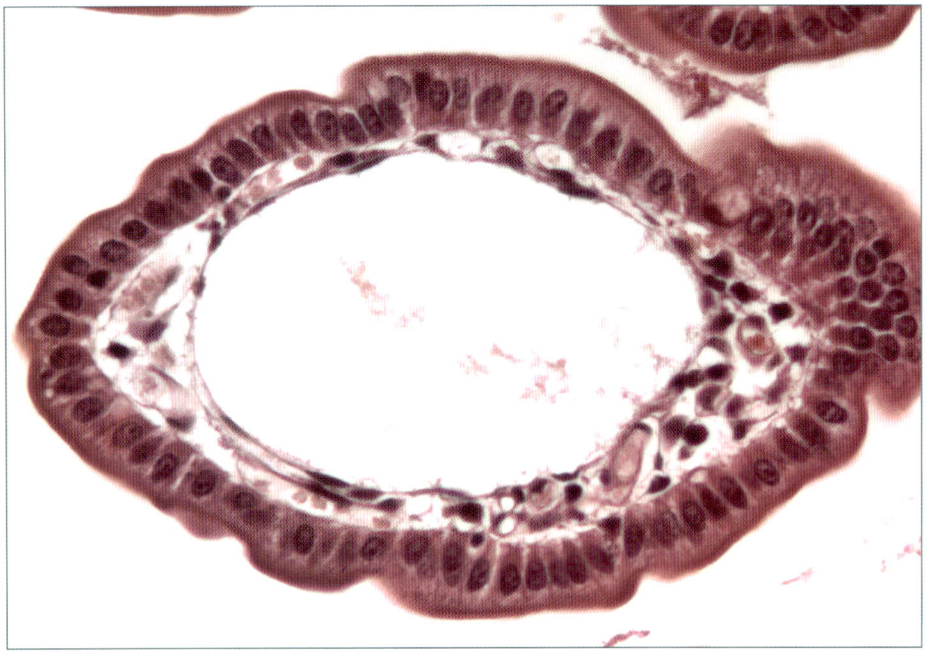

077 Thrombosis.
Coagulated mass occupying the lumen of a vessel in the intestinal submucosa in a case of typhlocolitis. HE.

078 Lymphangiectasia.
Dilatation of the central lacteal of an intestinal villus associated with alterations in mesenteric lymph drainage, including infectious lymphangitis. HE.

Inflammation

Inflammatory lesions of the intestine can be the manifestation of local or systemic processes. In mixed infections, included in the so-called enteric complex, lesions are the result of the concomitant pathogenic action of the agents involved. Enteritis, as used here, refers to inflammation of the small intestine. The terms typhlitis, colitis, and proctitis are reserved for inflammation of the large intestine.

Acute catarrhal inflammation

This section includes acute inflammatory lesions with few morphological alterations and those that involve shortening of the villi (atrophic inflammatory lesions).

079 Catarrhal enteritis.
Dilated, flaccid, translucent small intestine with aqueous contents. Suckling pig.

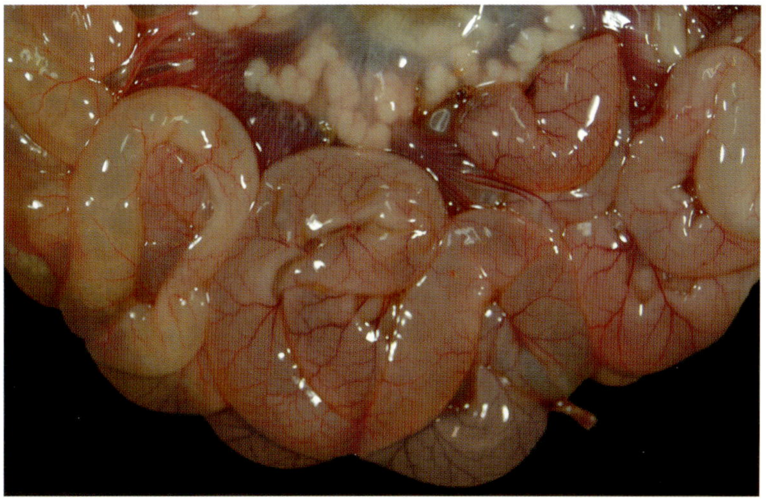

079

080 Catarrhal enteritis: atrophic form.
Thinning of the wall of the small intestine caused by a decrease in the height of the villi in a fixed sample. Suckling pig.

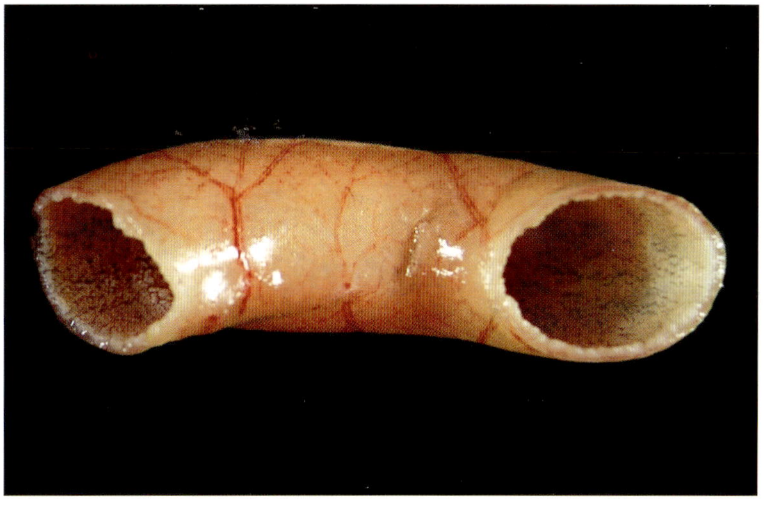

080

Lesion appearance can vary in different intestinal sections (e.g. in the case of viral infections).

081A

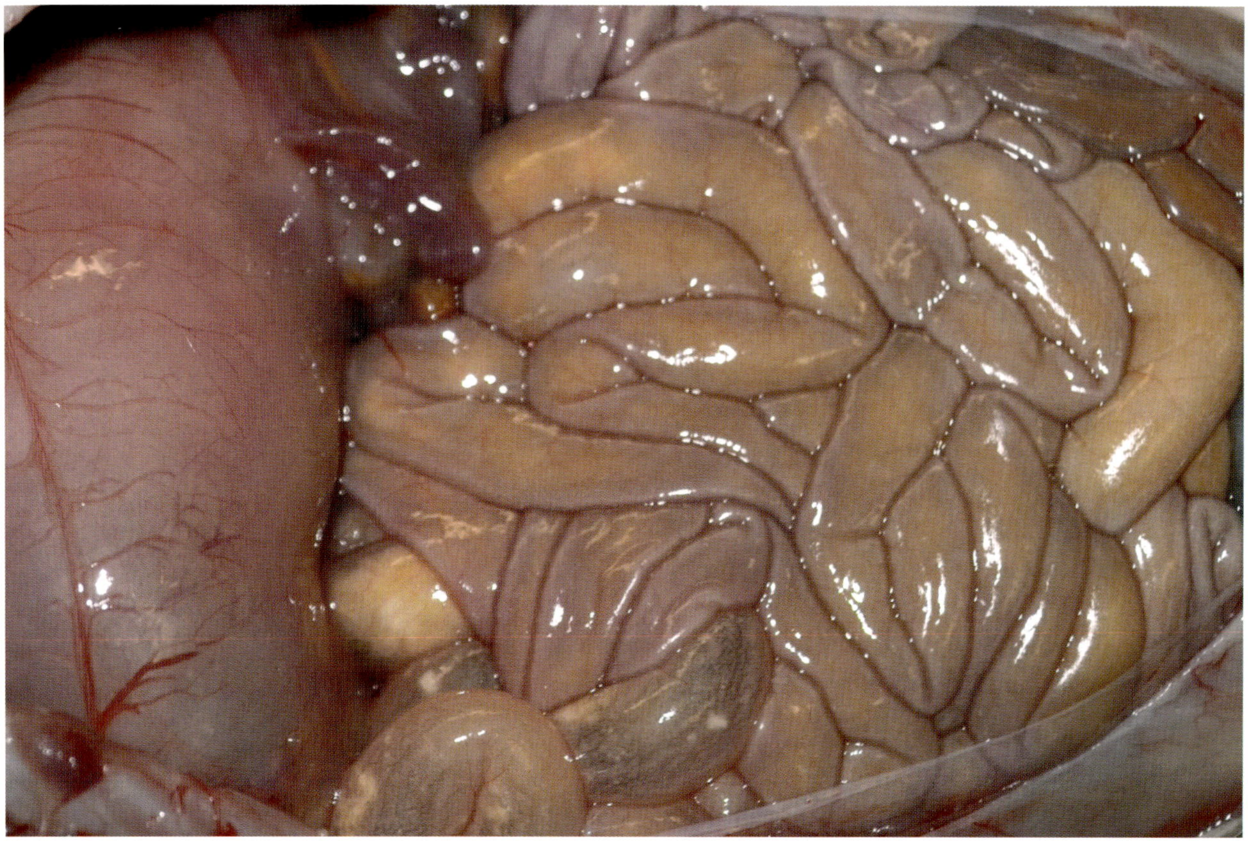

081A Catarrhal enteritis: atrophic form.
Dilated, thin-walled loops of the small intestine, which contains excess fluid content. Suckling pig.

081B

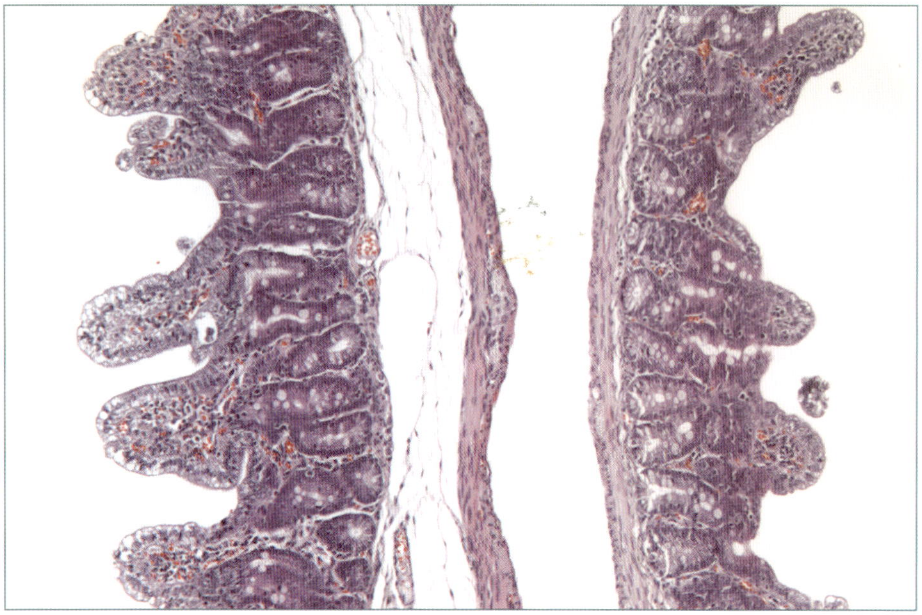

081B
Catarrhal enteritis: atrophic form.
Villi in two intestinal segments that are shortened and fused to varying degrees. Note the disproportion between the height of the villi and the depth of the crypts. HE.

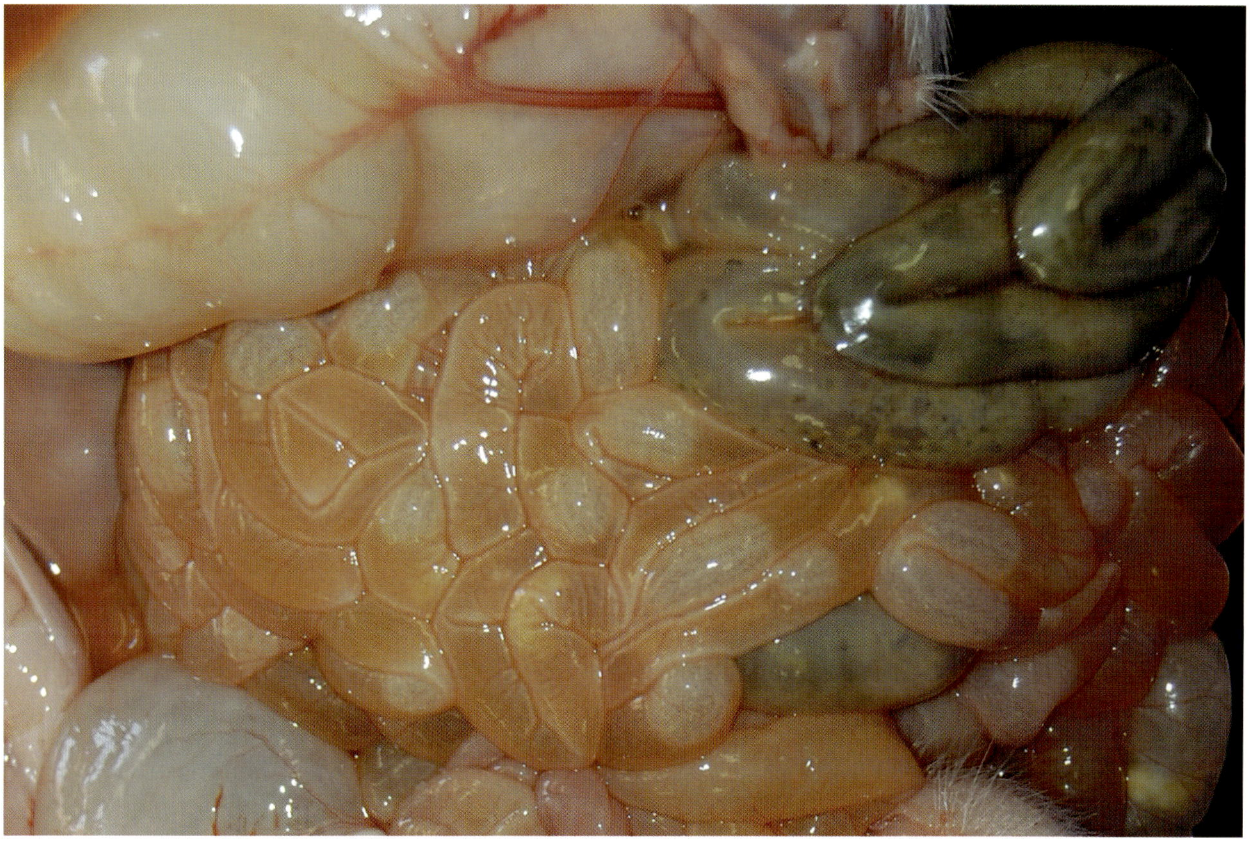

082A Catarrhal enteritis: atrophic form.
Flaccid, thin-walled small intestine with aqueous contents. Suckling pig.

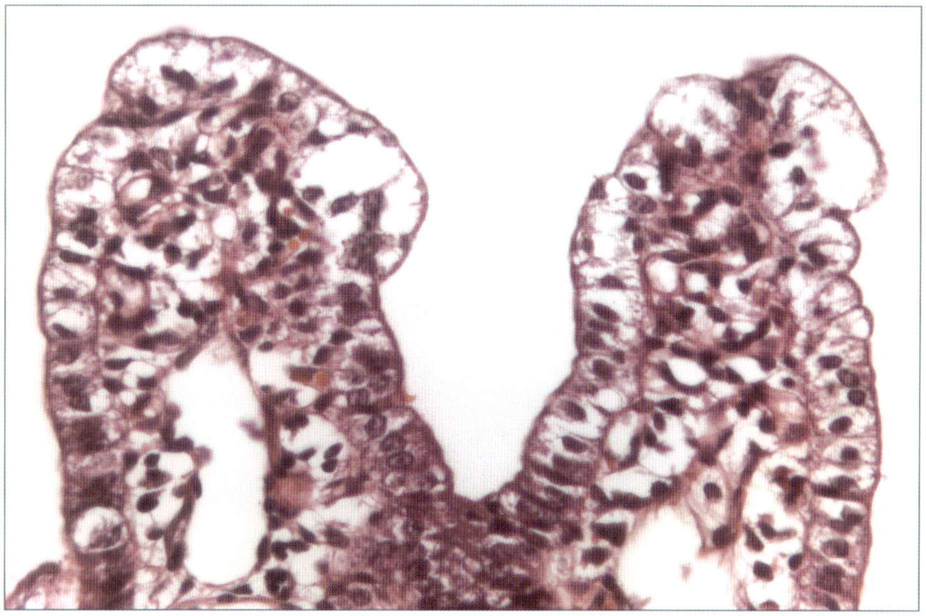

082B
Catarrhal enteritis: atrophic form.
Shortened and laterally fused villi, with vacuolisation of apical enterocytes. HE.

083A

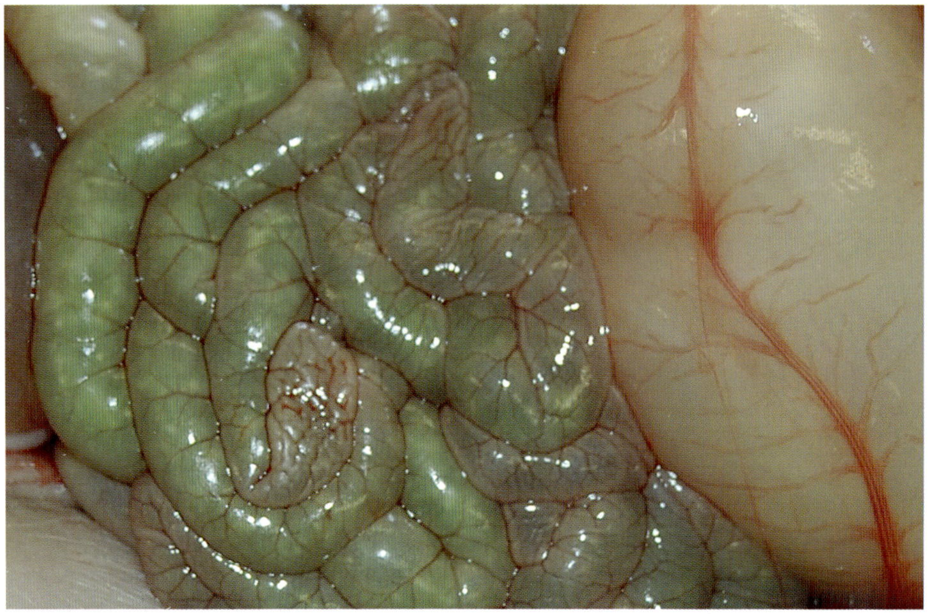

083B

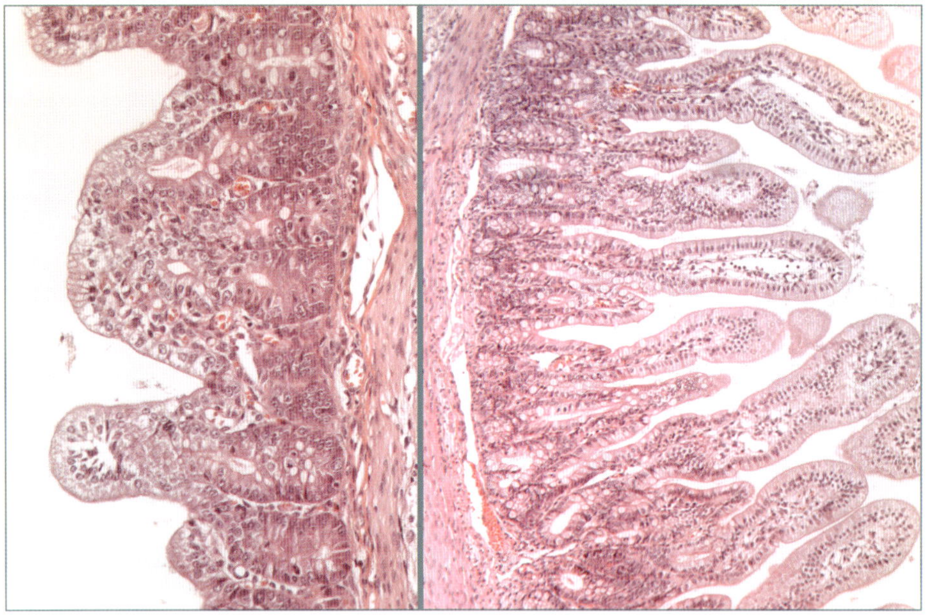

083A Catarrhal enteritis: atrophic form.
Dilation and generalised loss of tone of the small intestine. Suckling pig.

083B Catarrhal enteritis: atrophic form.
Shortened and fused villi in an intestinal segment (left), compared with the villi of another non-affected section (right). HE.

084A Catarrhal enteritis: atrophic form.
Reddened, flaccid, thin-walled small intestine containing a large volume of liquid. Suckling pig.

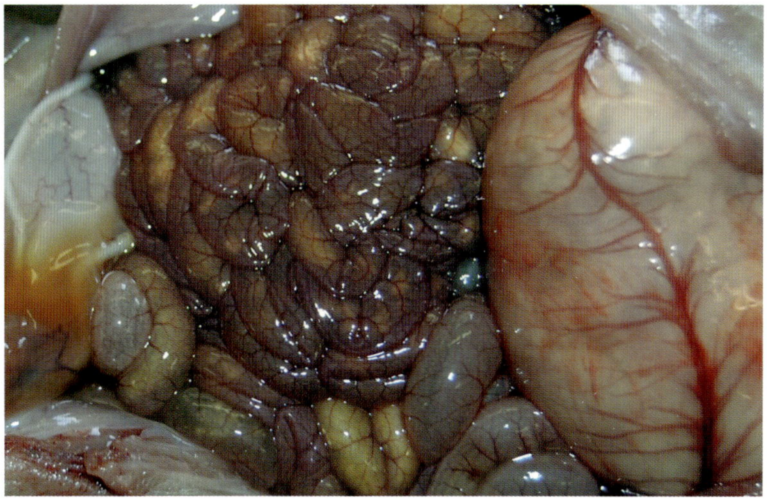

084A

084B Catarrhal enteritis: atrophic form.
Shortened, blunted, and fused villi (left) compared with those of a non-affected intestinal section (right). HE.

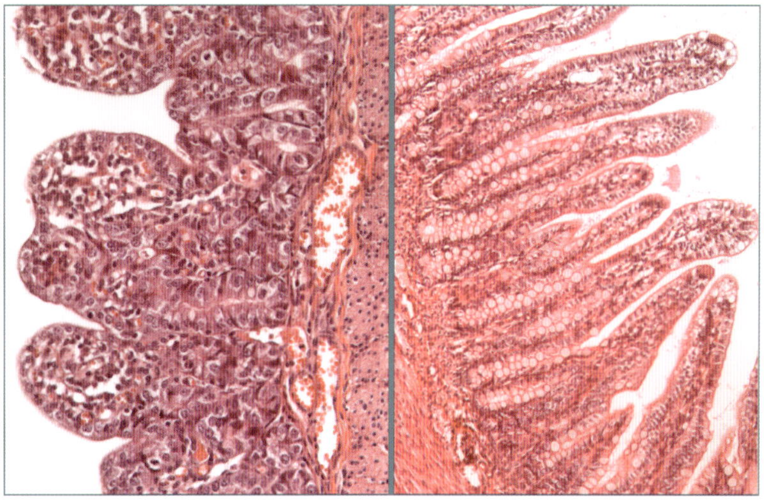

084B

084C Catarrhal enteritis: atrophic form.
Shortened and fused villi covered with flat cuboidal cells (left). Degeneration and flattening of the enterocytes of the apex of an intestinal villus (right). HE.

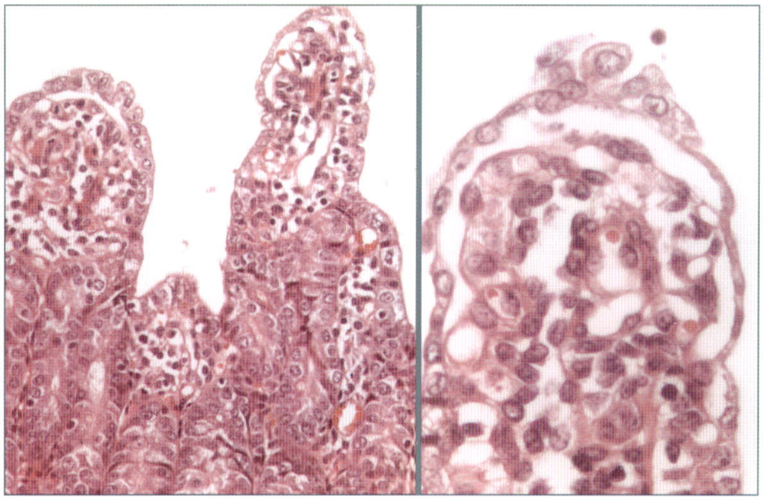

084C

085A

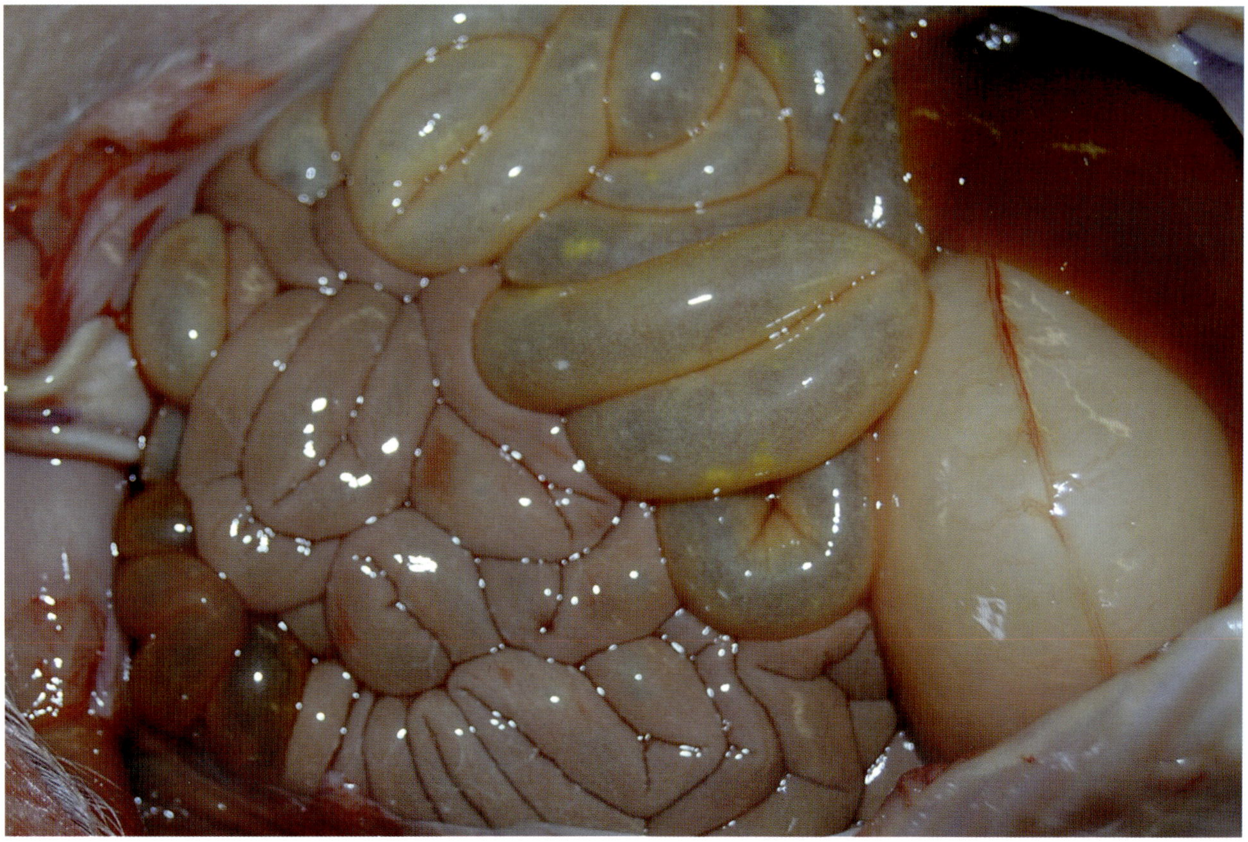

085A Catarrhal enteritis: atrophic form.
Thinning and dilation of the small intestine wall is more evident in certain intestinal sections with increased gas content. Suckling pig.

085B

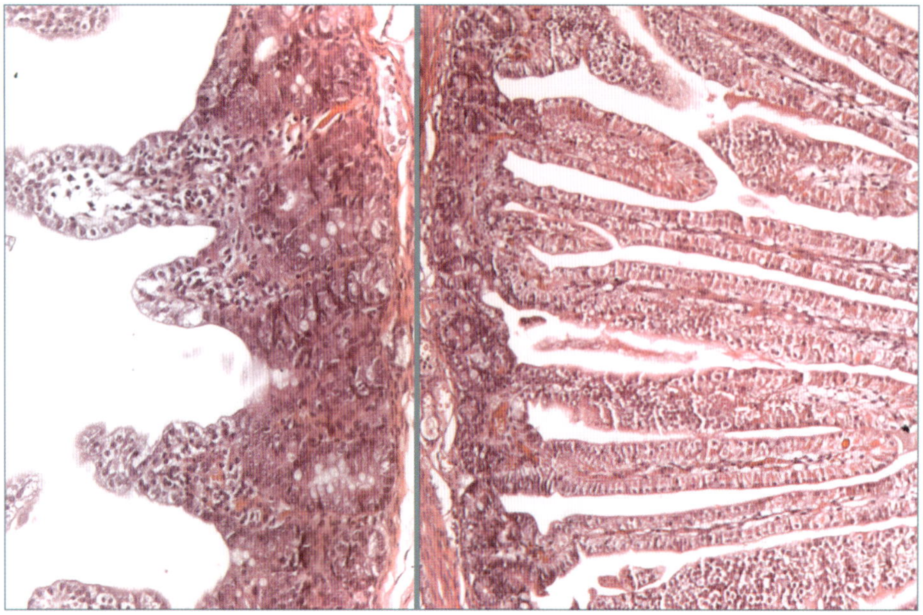

085B Catarrhal enteritis: atrophic form.
Uneven shortening of villi in a jejunal segment (left). Villi of another intestinal segment displaying no notable alterations (right). HE.

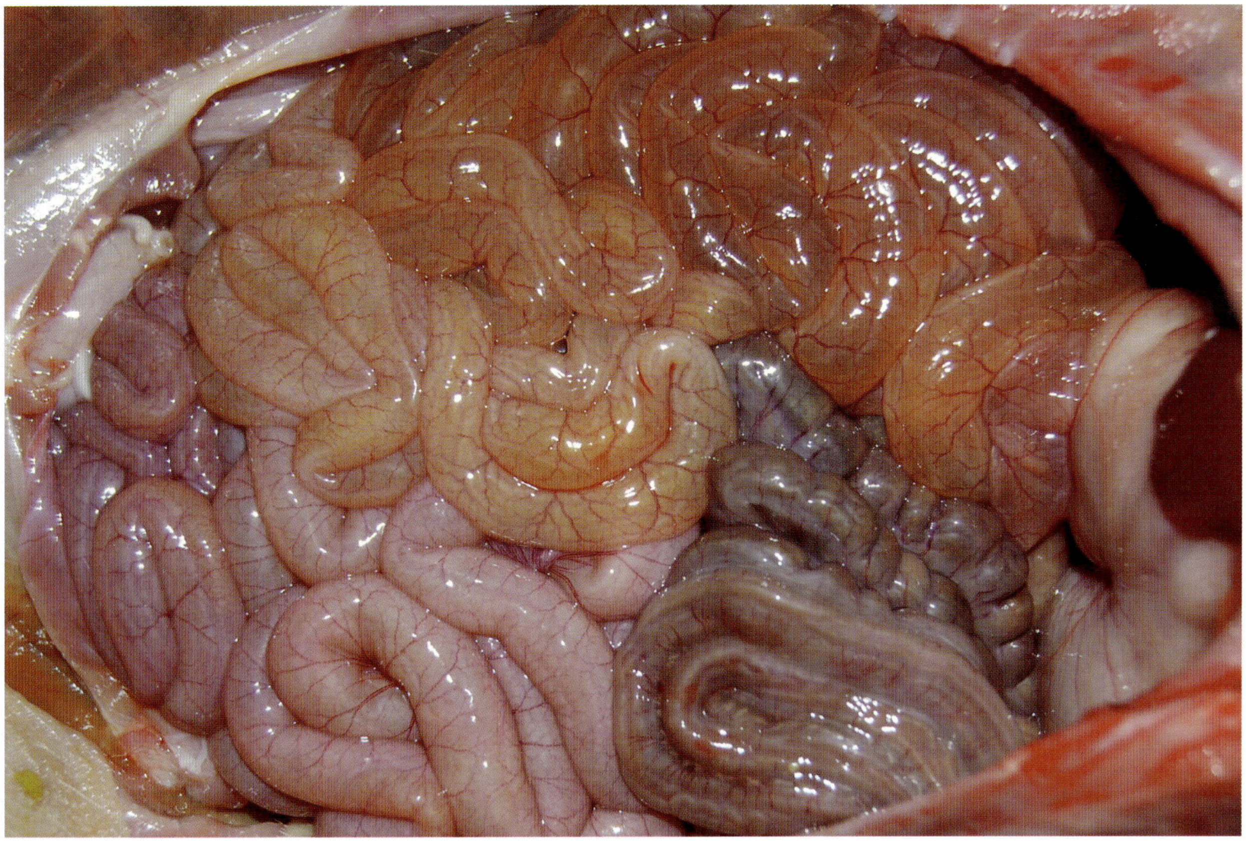

086A Catarrhal enteritis: atrophic form.

Small intestine displaying irregular flaccidity and alterations in colour due to the discontinuous nature of the lesions. The thinning of the wall is more evident in certain sections. Suckling pig.

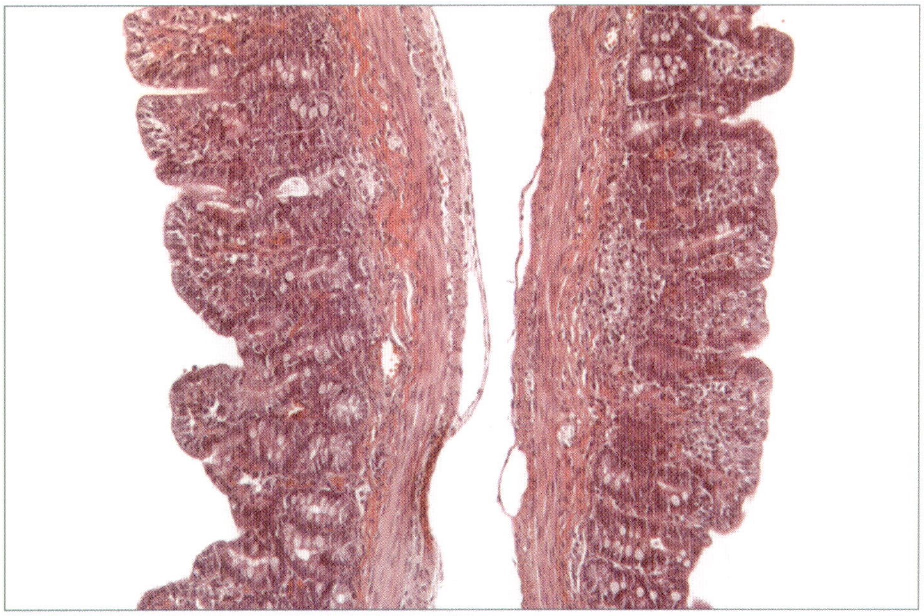

086B
Catarrhal enteritis: atrophic form.
Markedly shortened, blunted, and fused villi in two intestinal segments. HE.

087A

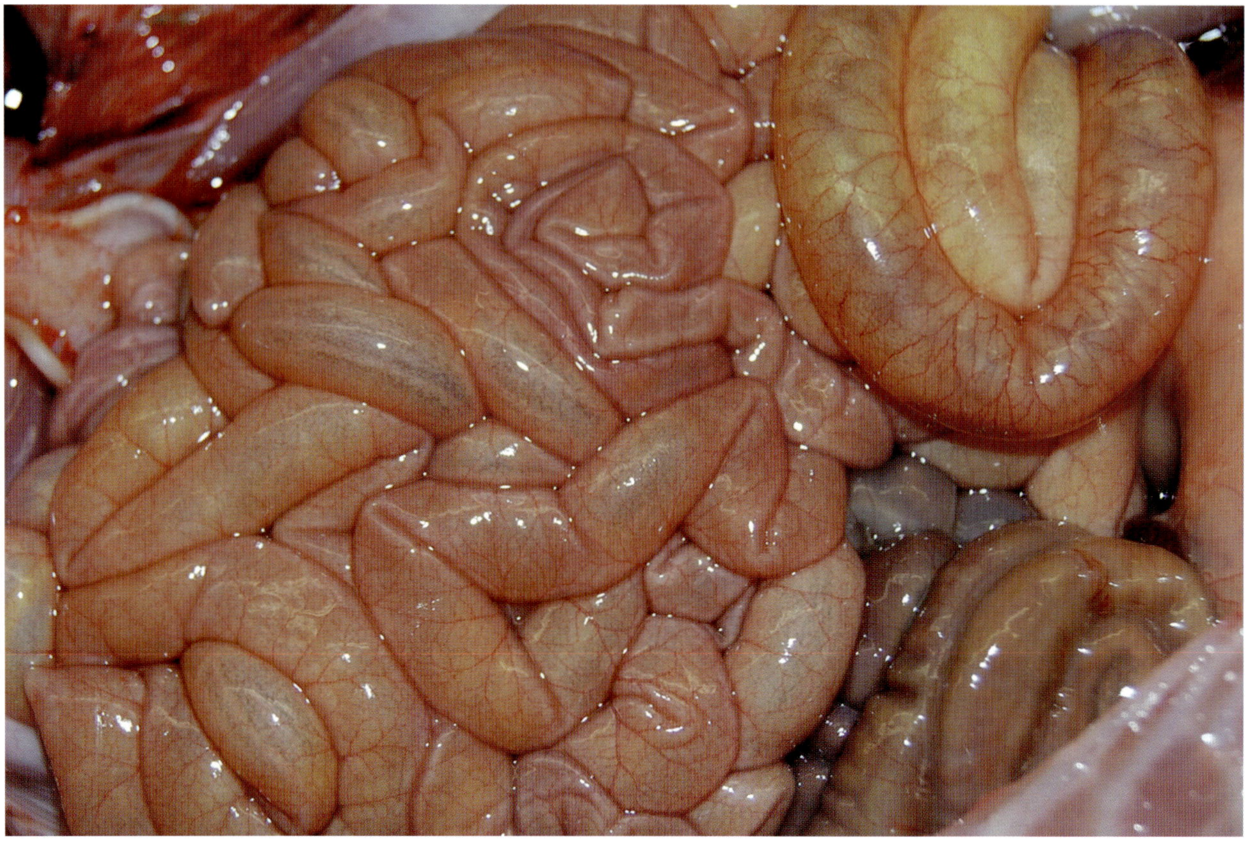

087A Catarrhal enteritis: atrophic form.
Flaccid small intestine exhibiting diffuse dilation. Suckling pig.

087B

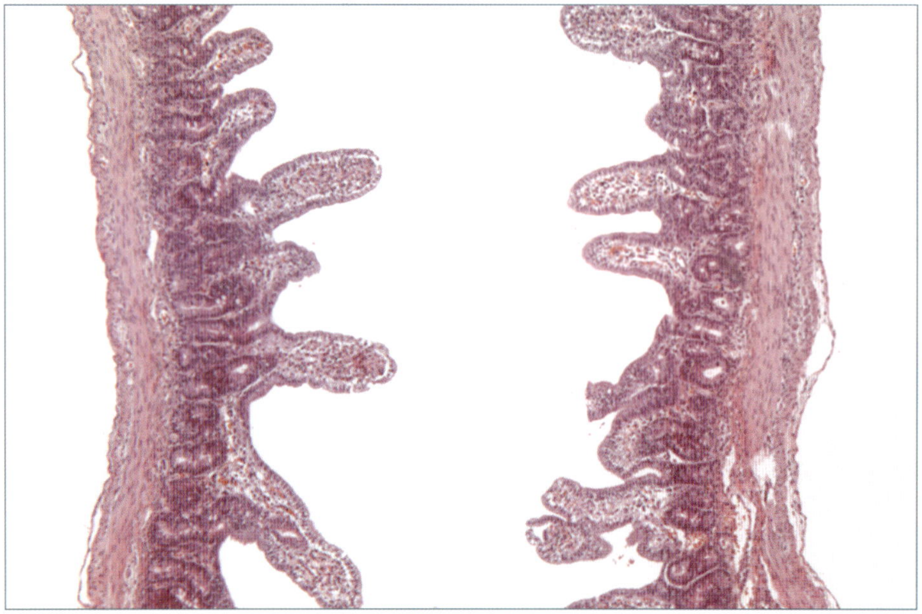

087B
Catarrhal enteritis: atrophic form.
Uneven shortening of the villi along the entire length of the intestinal segment. HE.

088A

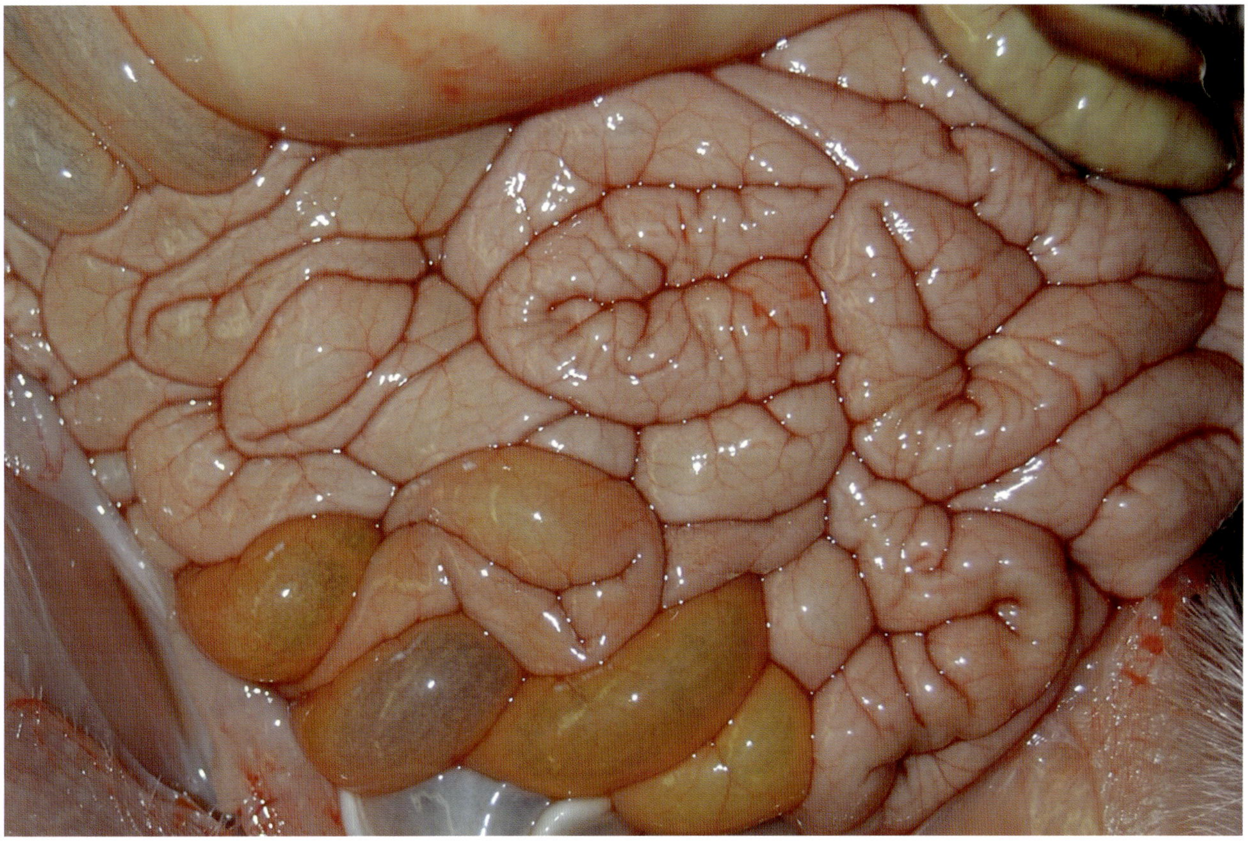

088A Catarrhal enteritis: atrophic form.
Diffuse dilatation and loss of tone of the loops of the small intestine. Suckling pig.

088B

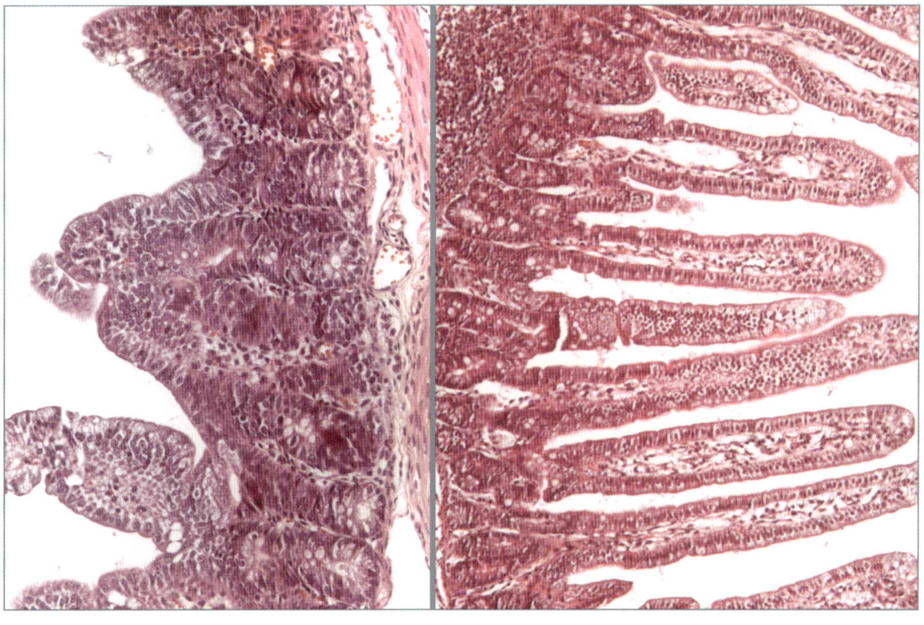

088B
Catarrhal enteritis: atrophic form.
Shortening and fusion of the villi (left). Villi in a section of unaffected intestine (right). HE.

089A

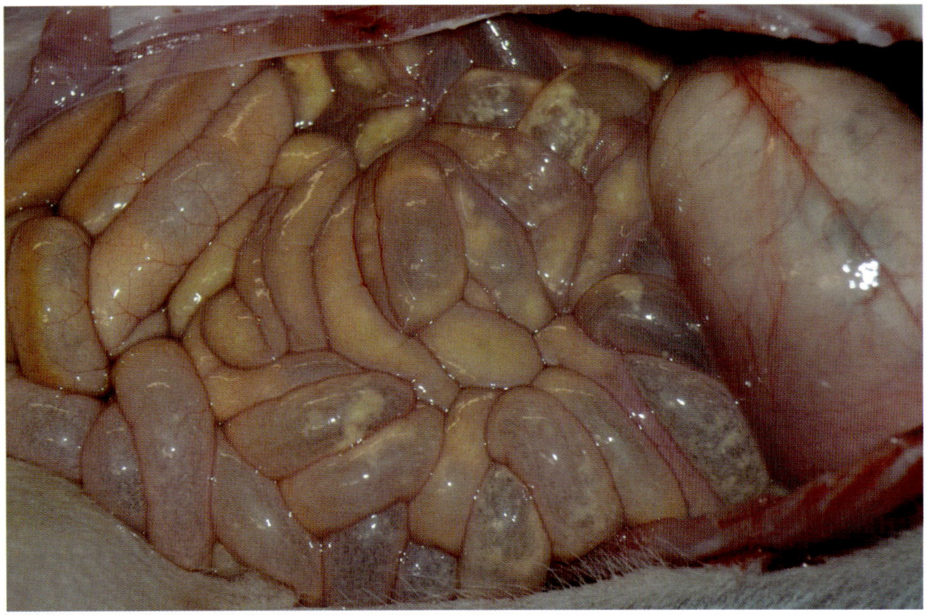

089A

Catarrhal enteritis: atrophic form.

Dilation, flaccidity, and parietal thinning of the loops of the small intestine. Suckling pig.

089B

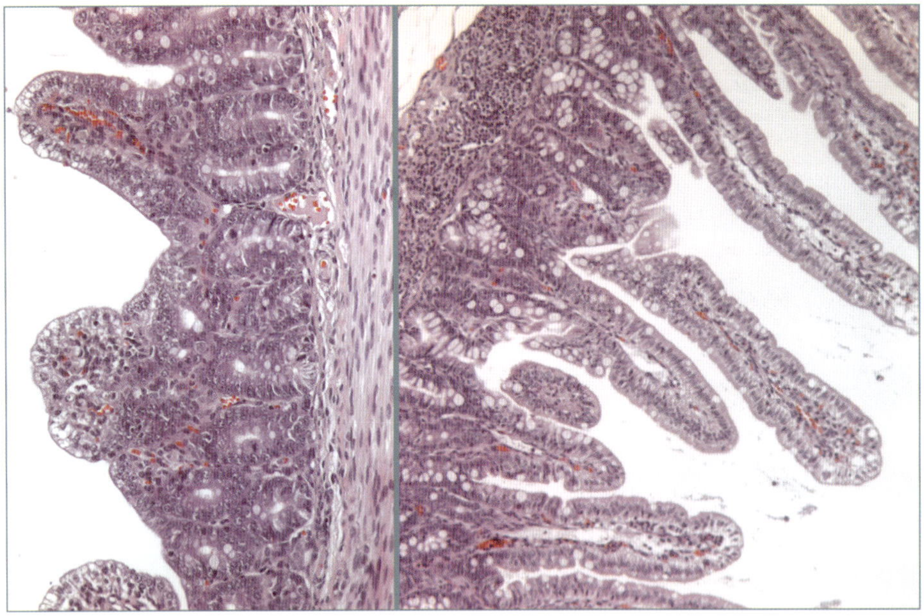

089B

Catarrhal enteritis: atrophic form.

Shortened and fused villi of a jejunal segment (left) compared with those of an unaffected segment (right). HE.

Villous atrophy with compensatory crypt hyperplasia is characteristic of catarrhal enteritis in suckling piglets, linked to the pathogenic action of coronaviruses and rotaviruses. Atrophic lesions caused by coccidia are shown in the corresponding section.

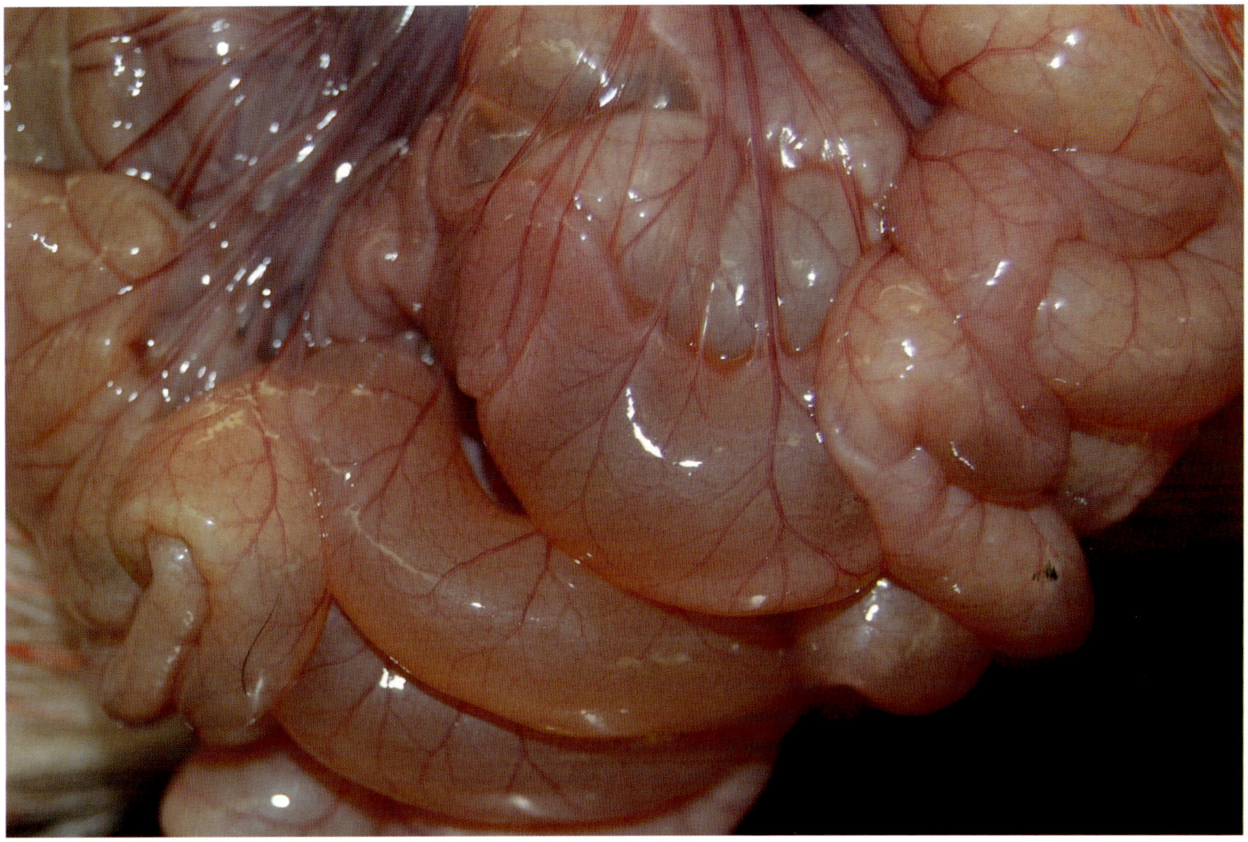

090A

090A Catarrhal enteritis: atrophic form.
Some loops of the small intestine are more dilated and translucent than others. Suckling pig.

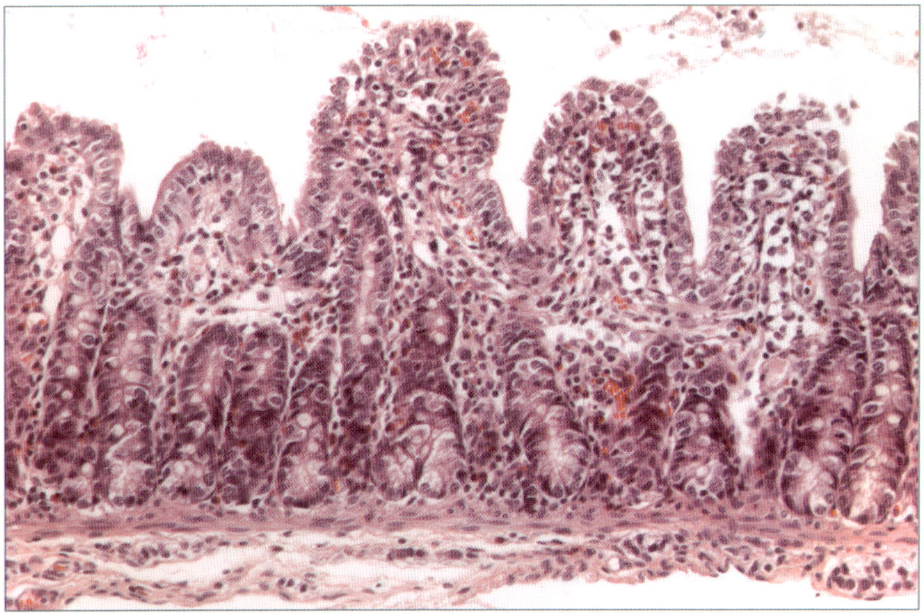

090B

090B
Catarrhal enteritis: atrophic form.
Intestinal segment showing retracted villi, with desquamation of apical enterocytes. HE.

091

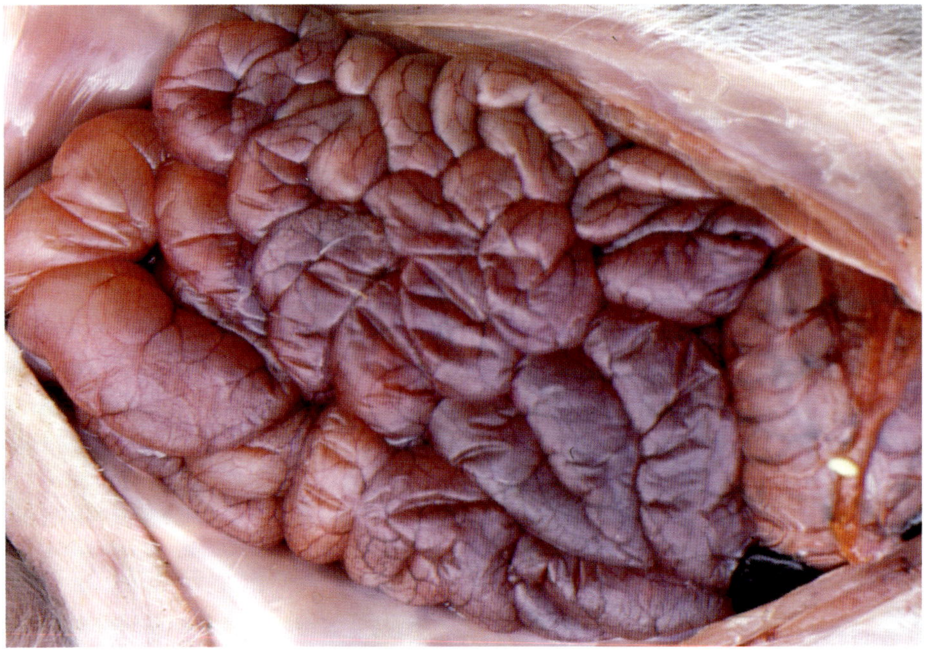

092

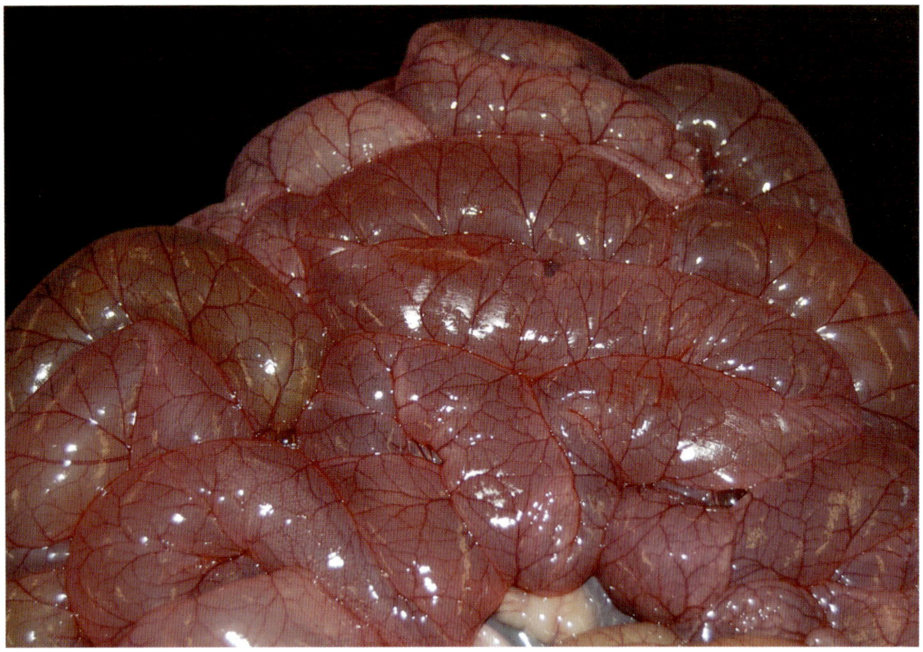

091 Catarrhal enteritis.
Intestinal loops displaying diffuse reddening, dilation, and flaccidity. Weaner pig.

092 Catarrhal enteritis.
Expansion and increased colouration of the loops of the small intestine. Weaner pig.

093A Catarrhal enteritis.

Some segments of the small intestine are thin-walled and flaccid. Others appear paler and bloated. Weaner pig.

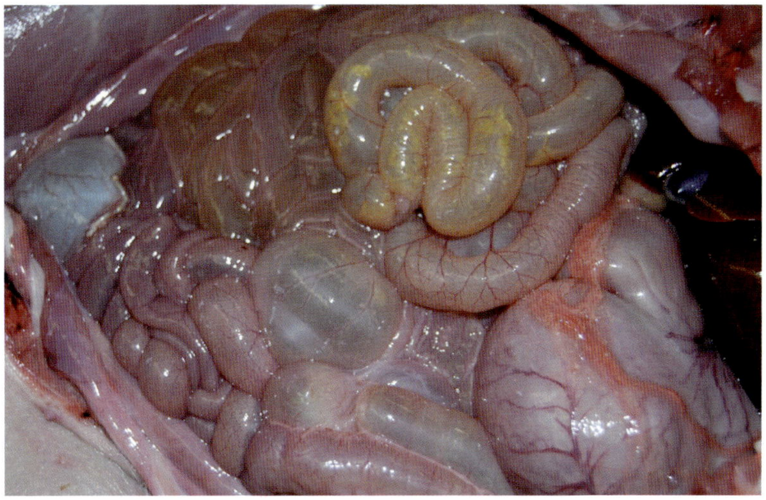
093A

093B Catarrhal enteritis.

Dilated blood vessels in the submucosa displaying leukocyte margination. HE.

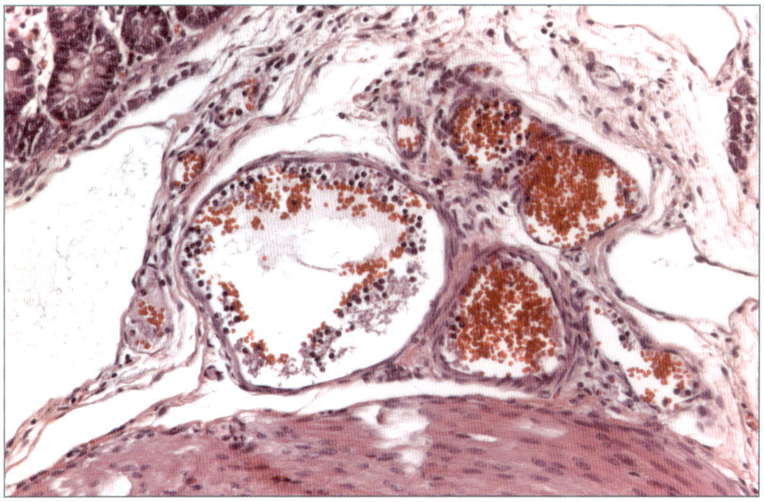
093B

093C Catarrhal enteritis.

Villus with no evident epithelial alterations, but displaying a marked increase in neutrophils in the capillaries of the lamina propria (left). Bacterial adhesion to the enterocytes of a villus (right). HE.

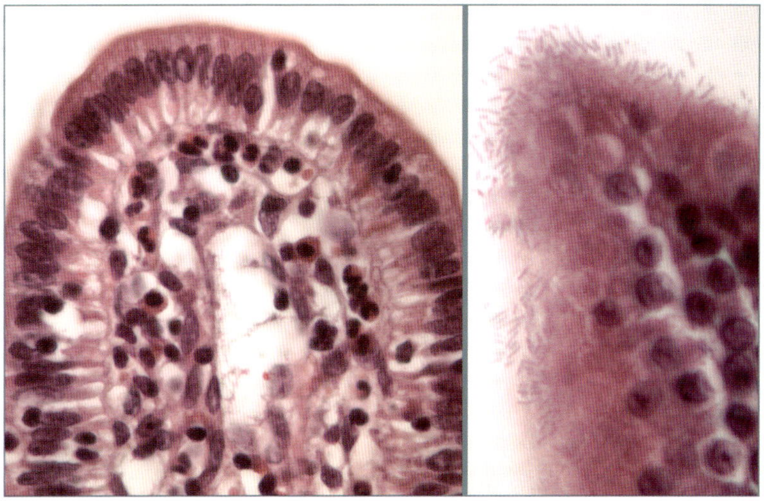
093C

094A

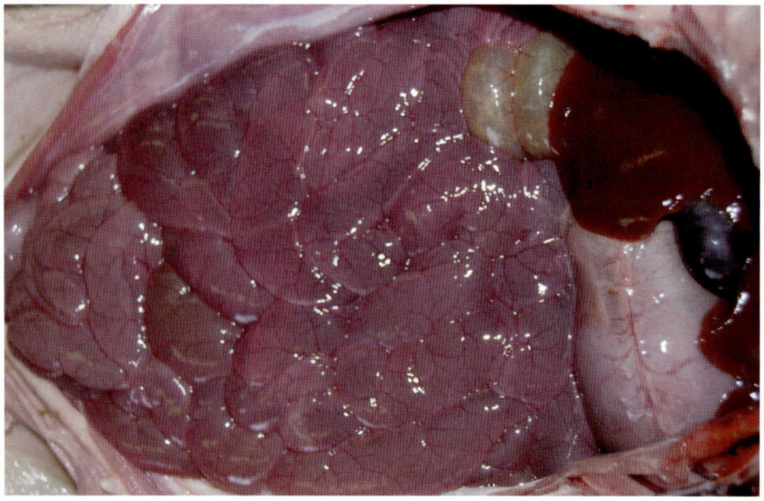

094A Catarrhal enteritis.
Small intestine showing diffuse reddening, flaccidity, and dilation. Weaner pig.

094B

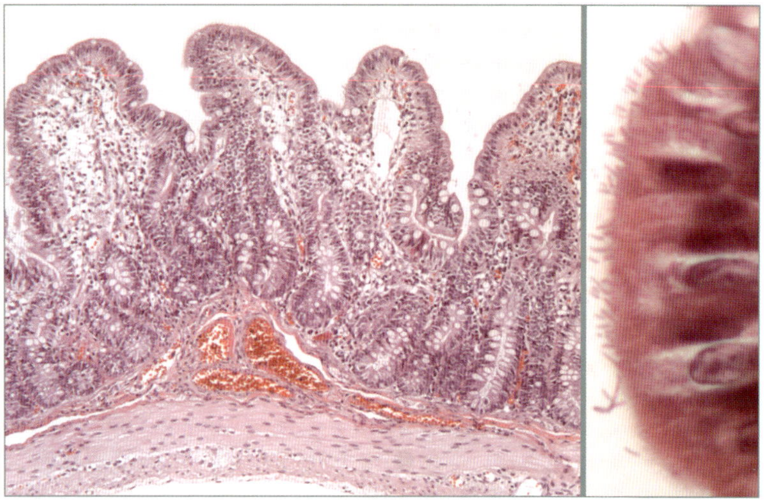

094B Catarrhal enteritis.
Hyperaemia of the lamina propria and submucosa with general conservation of the structure of the villi (left). Bacterial adhesion to enterocytes (right). HE.

095A

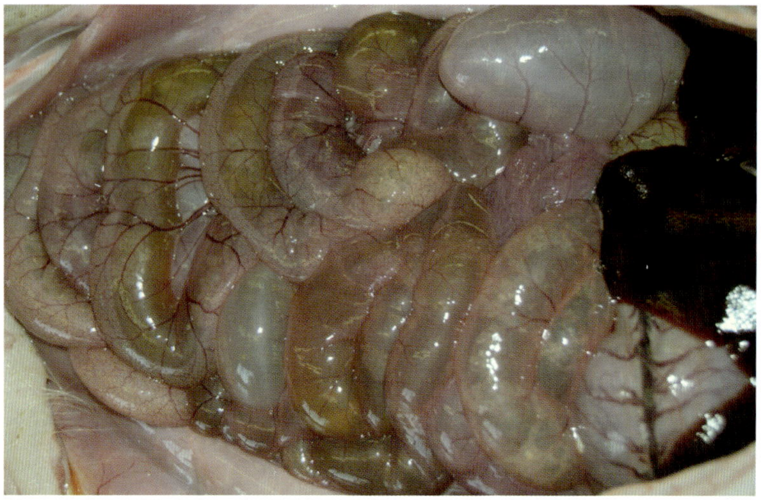

095A Catarrhal enteritis.
Generalised intestinal dilatation, prominent blood vessels, and variable increase in colour depending on content. Weaner pig.

095B **Catarrhal enteritis.**
Preservation of the integrity of the villous epithelium (left) with bacterial adhesion to the surface of enterocytes (right). HE.

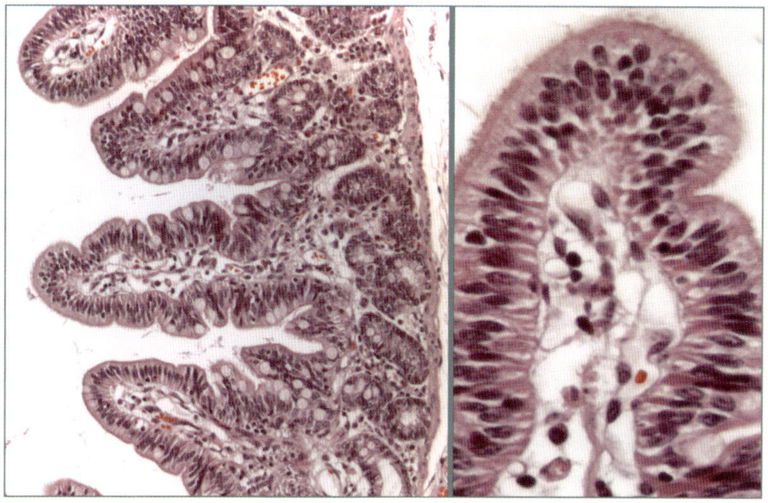

095B

096 **Bacterial adhesion.**
Layer of microbes on the surface of the enterocytes of the villi in a case of catarrhal enteritis. Weaner pig. HE.

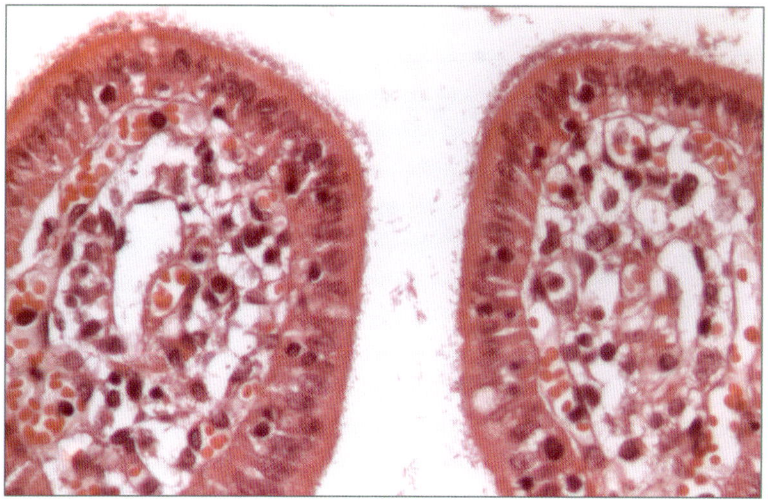

096

Lesions in catarrhal enteritis caused by colibacillosis infection in suckling and weaner pigs are not specific. Histopathology shows bacterial adhesion to enterocytes, hyperaemia, and increased numbers of neutrophils in the lamina propria. Epithelial alterations are not significant, and villous atrophy, if present, is usually mild.

Haemorrhagic inflammation

This form involves extravasation of erythrocytes due to vascular damage, together with other inflammatory intestinal alterations.

097

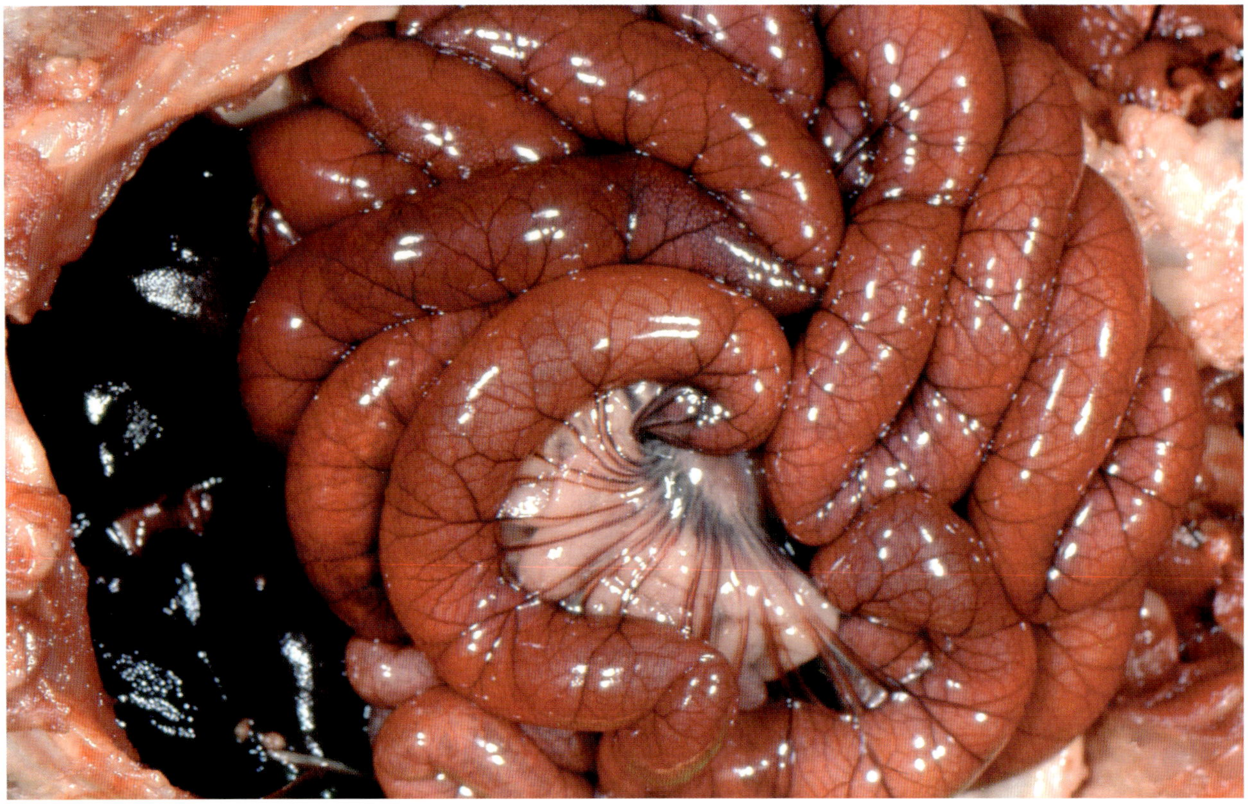

097 **Haemorrhagic enteritis.**
Diffuse reddening of the small intestine. Weaner pig.

098

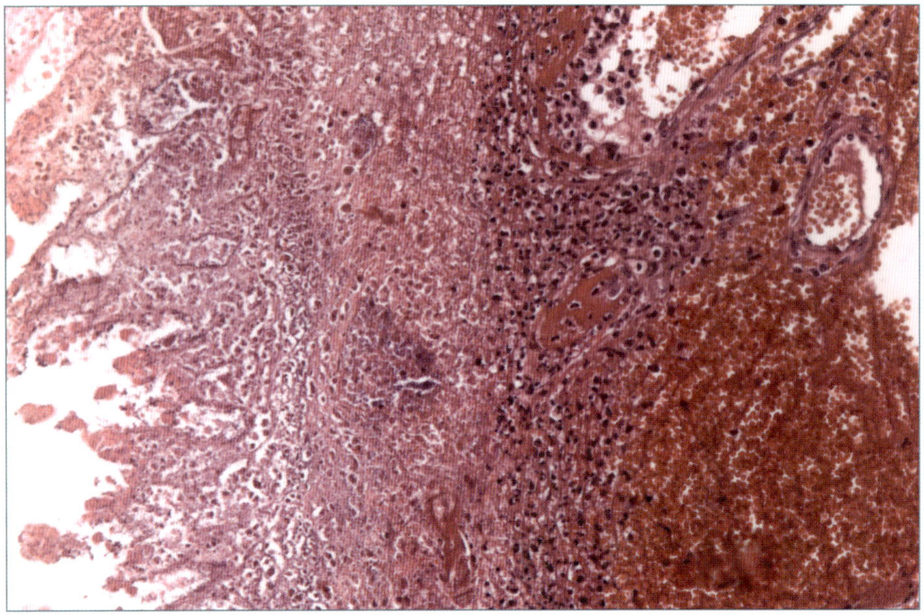

098 **Haemorrhagic enteritis.**
Blood extravasation in the wall of the small intestine with concomitant mucosal necrosis. Suckling pig.

099 **Haemorrhagic enteritis.** Leukocytic infiltration and extravasation of erythrocytes in the lamina propria of the small intestine. Fattening pig.

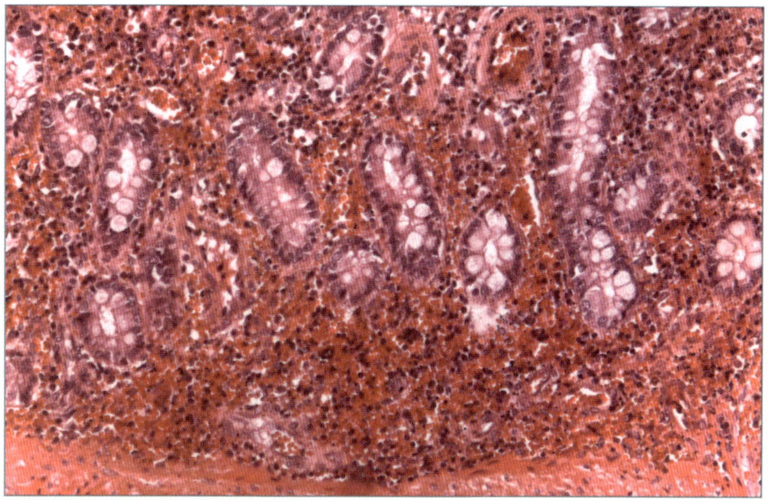

099

100 **Haemorrhagic colitis.** Deep red mucosa in two segments of the large intestine with dark-coloured foci. Fattening pig.

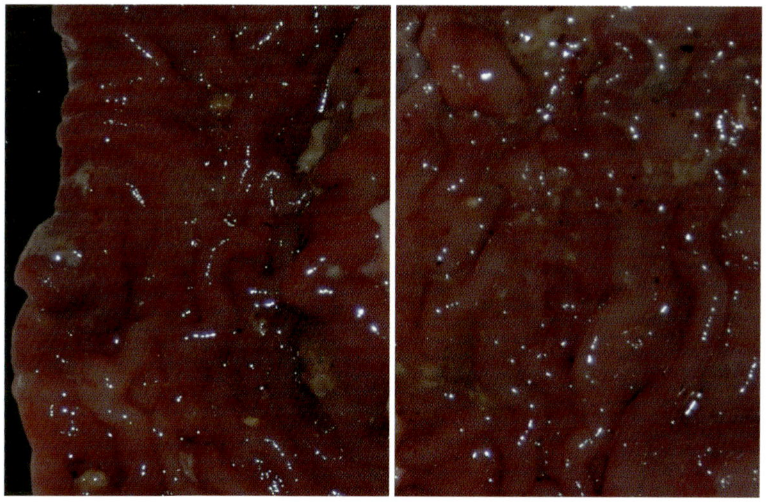

100

Haemorrhagic intestinal inflammation is associated with *Clostridium perfringens* type C infection in suckling pigs. In other production phases this condition can be found associated with haemorrhagic *E. coli* gastroenteritis, dysentery, septicaemic salmonellosis, proliferative enteritis, and trichuriasis, often in the fibrinohaemorrhagic form.

Fibrinous inflammation

In this inflammatory process fibrin constitutes an important component of the exudate, although other constituents may also be present. The fibrinous exudate can form a lamina or pseudomembrane over the intestinal mucosa. Two types of fibrinous pseudomembranous inflammation are described: non-necrotising (croupy) and necrotising (diphtheroid). The use of this expression to describe cases in which the lamina is formed by necrotic mucosa is a matter of debate.

101A

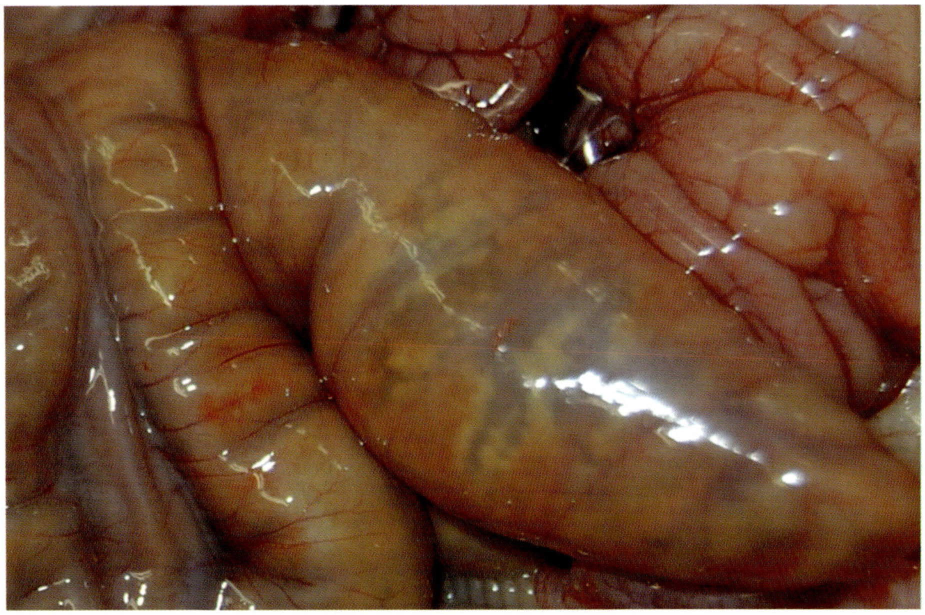

101A

Fibrinous typhlocolitis.
Pseudomembranes identifiable as yellowish plaques, visible through the serosa of the caecum. Suckling pig.

101B

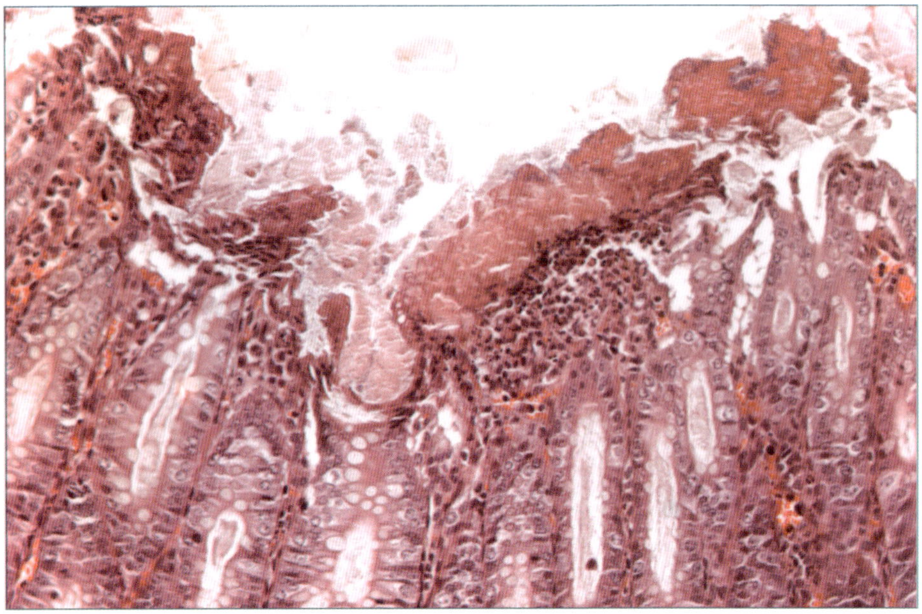

101B

Fibrinous typhlocolitis.
Exudate, consisting of fibrin, leukocytes, and mucus, on top of the eroded mucosa. Superficial lamina propria infiltrated by neutrophils. HE.

102A

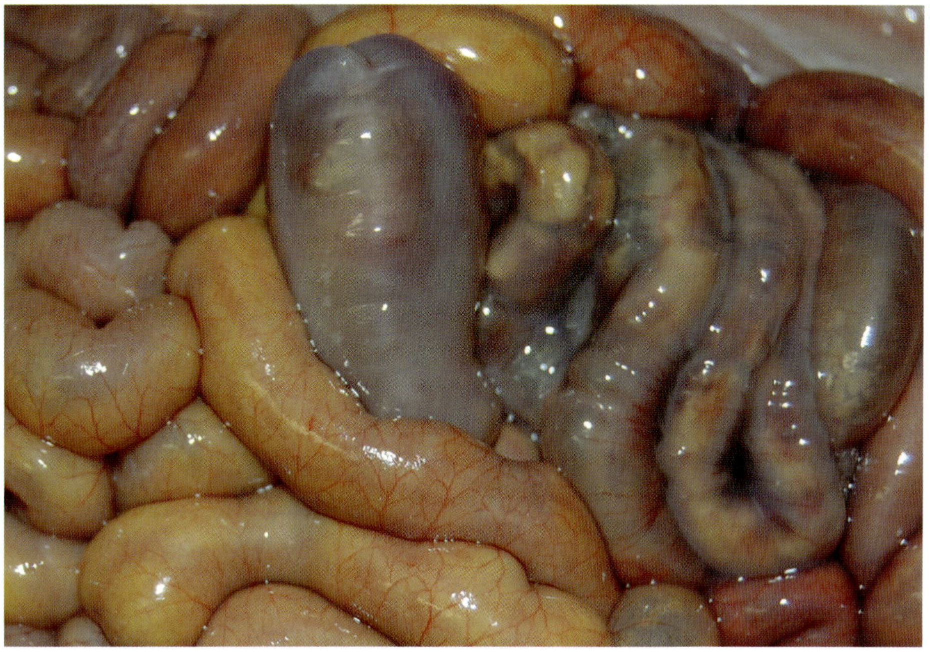

102B

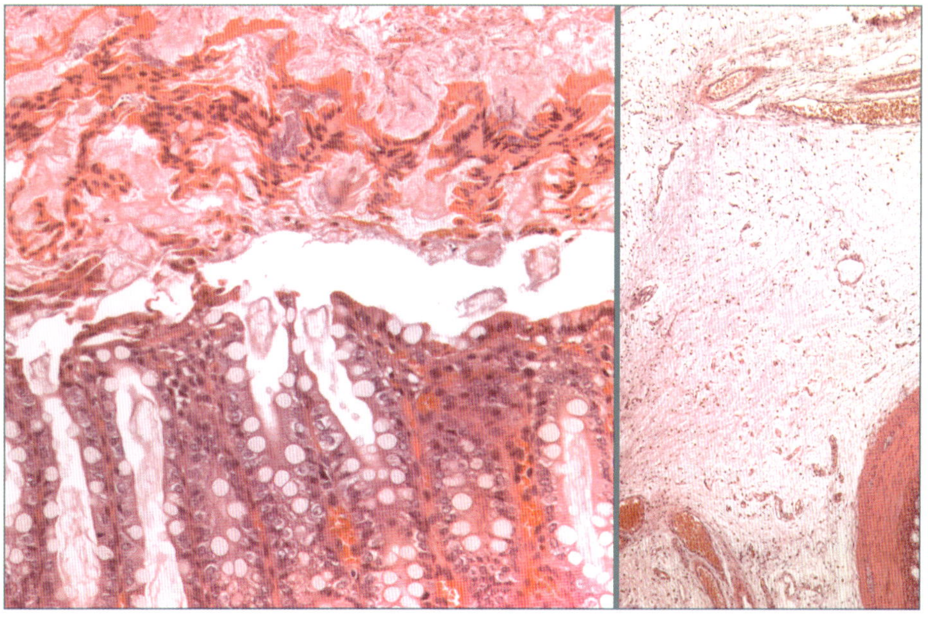

102A Fibrinous typhlocolitis.
Patchy appearance of large intestine due to the presence of pseudomembranes visible through the serosa in the form of yellowish plaques with reddish foci. Enlargement of the mesocolon due to oedema.
Suckling pig.

102B Fibrinous typhlocolitis.
Pseudomembrane composed of fibrin, epithelial cells, mucus, and leukocytes (left). Tissue expansion between loops of the colon consistent with concomitant oedema. HE.

103A

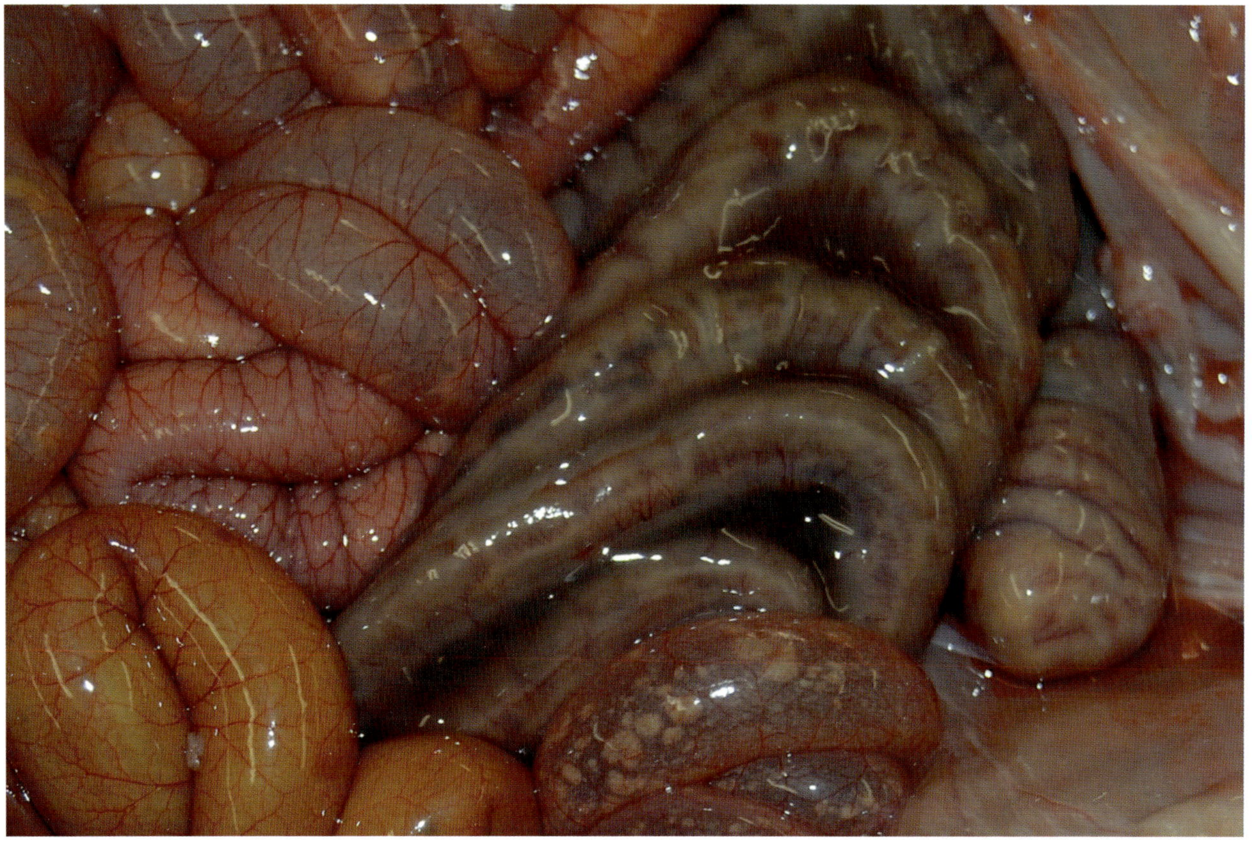

103A Fibrinous typhlocolitis.

Large intestine appears compact and the serosa has a reticulated appearance due to the presence of pseudomembranous deposits in the mucosa. Suckling pig.

103B

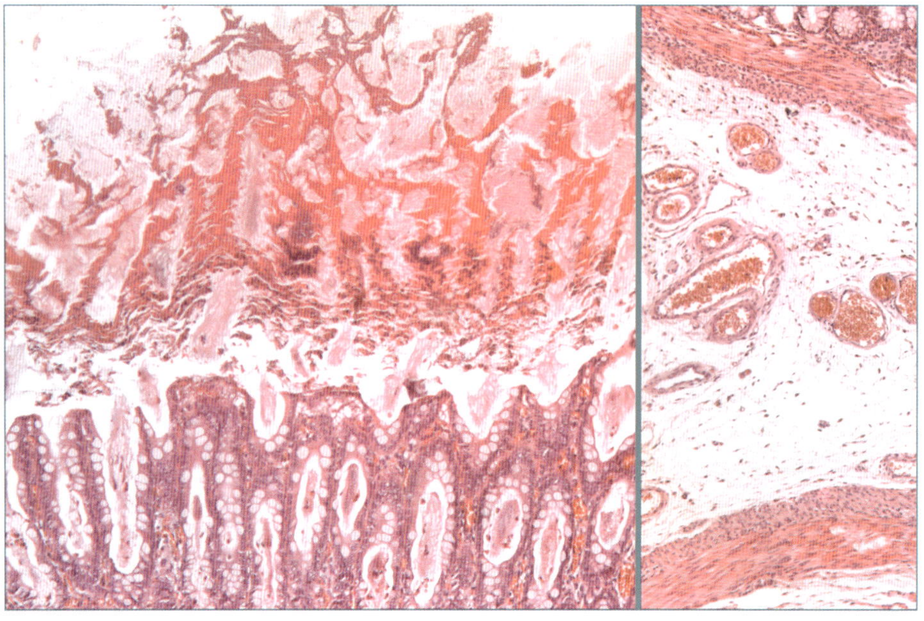

103B Fibrinous typhlocolitis.

Eruptive pseudomembranous exudate on the mucosa (left). Increased space and tissue pallor between two loops of the colon due to oedema associated with the process. HE.

104A

Fibrinous typhlocolitis.
The large intestine is swollen due to its pasty content, with a gelatinous film separating the loops of the colon. Suckling pig.

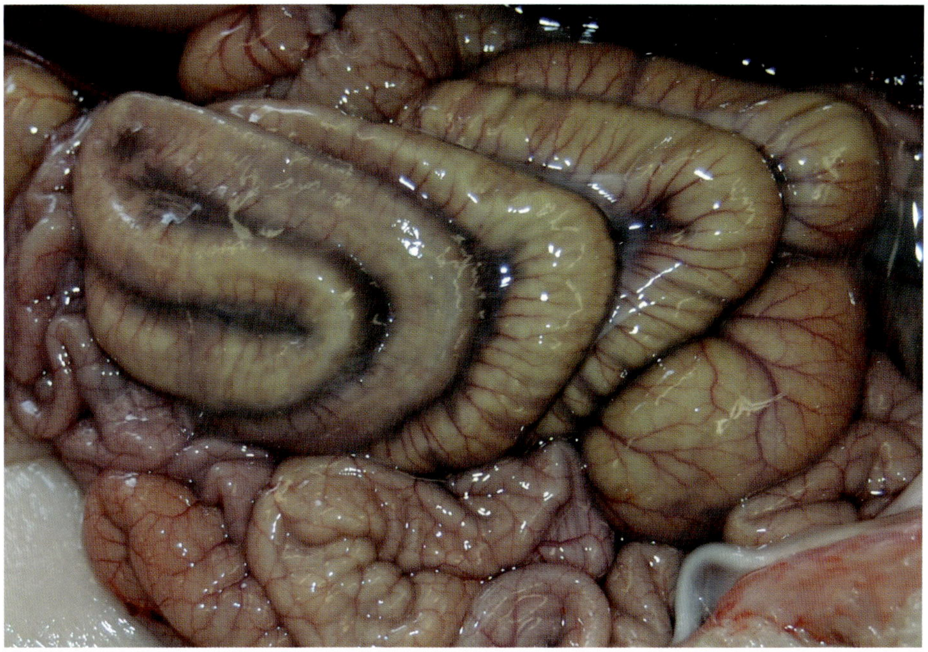

104A

104B

Fibrinous typhlocolitis.
Pseudomembranous exudate of fibrin, leukocytes, and cell debris on an eroded mucosal surface (left). Mesocolon oedema associated with inflammation, resulting in dilation of the space between two loops (right). HE.

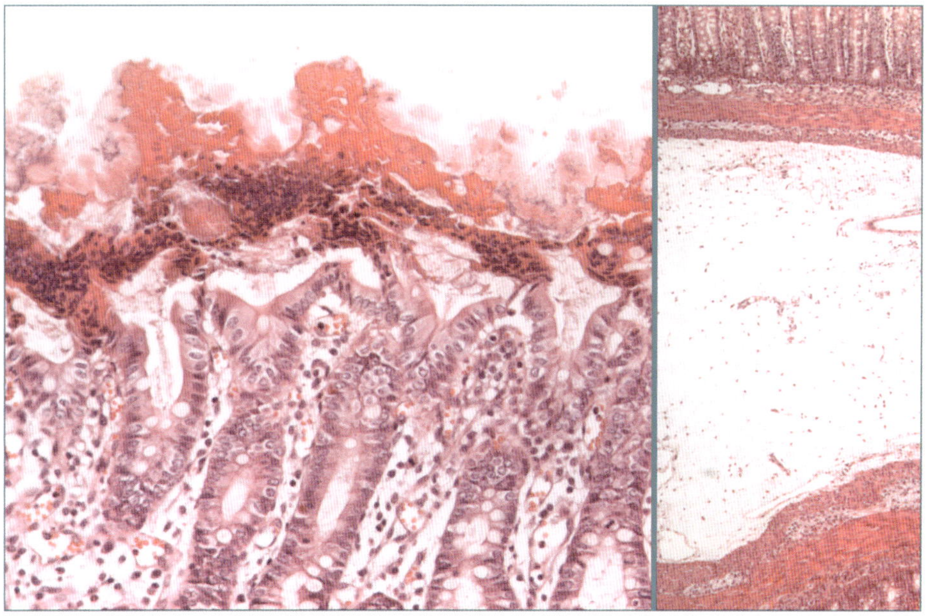

104B

Pseudomembranous typhlocolitis is associated with *Clostridium difficile* infection in piglets. Deep mucosal necrosis may be observed in some cases. Mesocolon oedema, which is characteristic of this process, is not considered pathognomonic.

105A

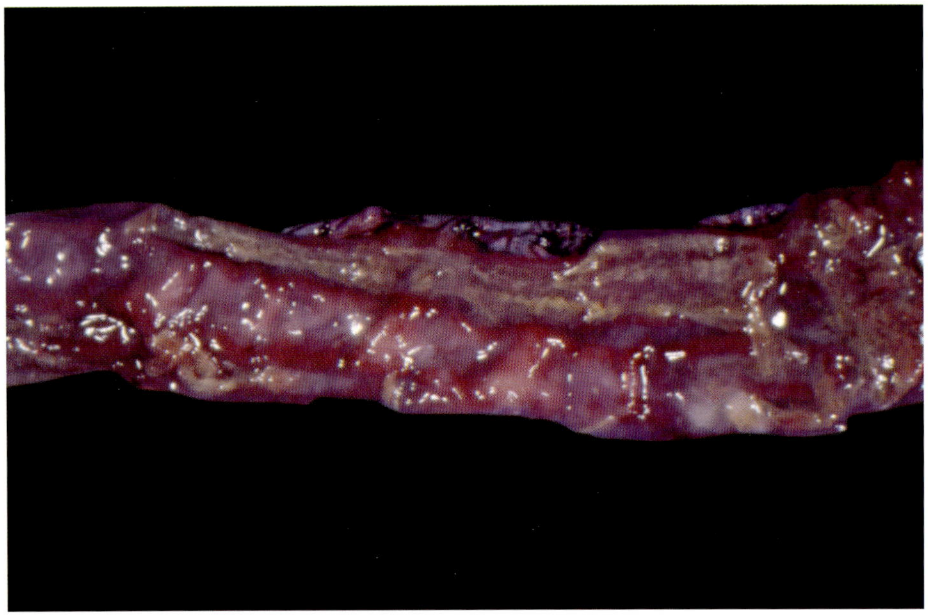

105B

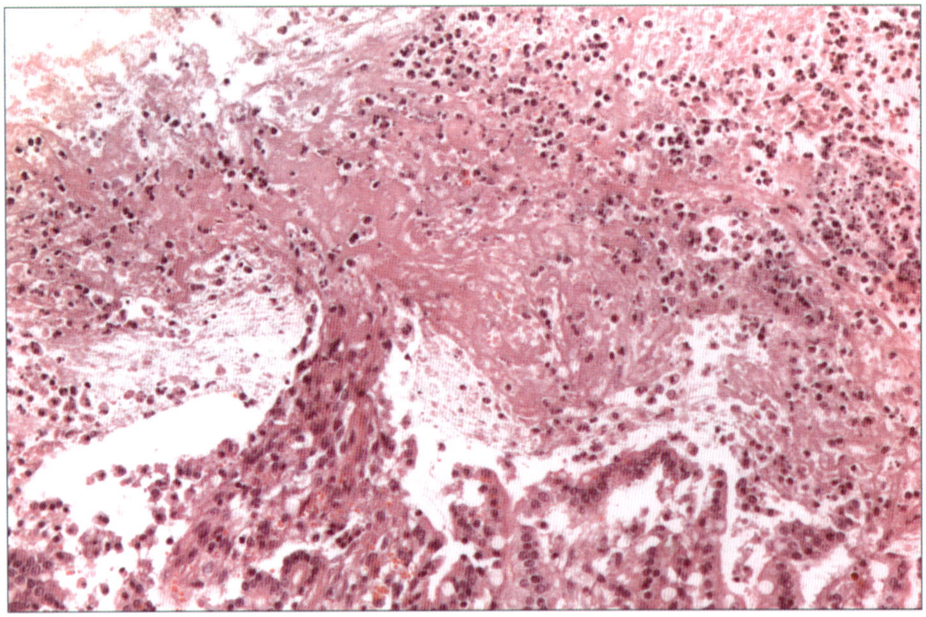

105A Fibrinous enteritis.
The mucosa of the small intestine is reddened with greyish, irregular-shaped adhesions that form longitudinal lines. Weaner pig.

105B Fibrinous enteritis.
Pseudomembranous exudate consisting of fibrin, leukocytes, and cell debris, with alteration of the mucosal surface. HE.

106A **Fibrinous enteritis.** Mucosa of the small intestine exhibiting thickened folds, covered with greyish velvet-like deposits. Fattening pig.

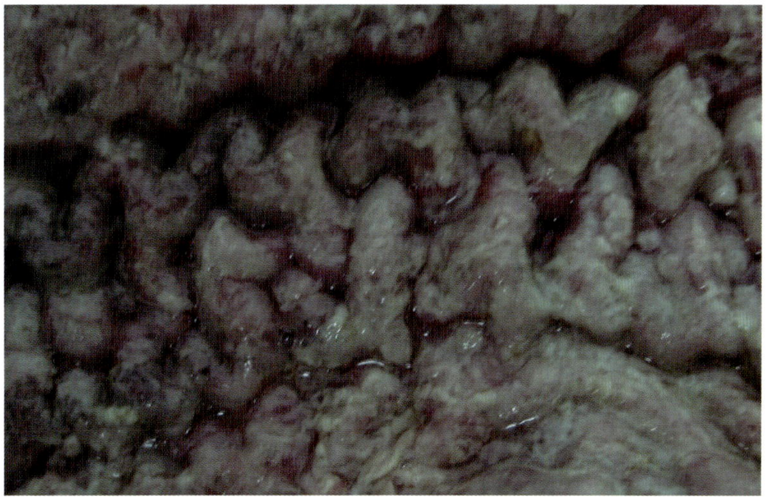

106A

106B **Fibrinous enteritis.** Exudate consisting of fibrin, leukocytes, and desquamated cells extending over the mucosa of the small intestine, which shows alterations at certain points. HE.

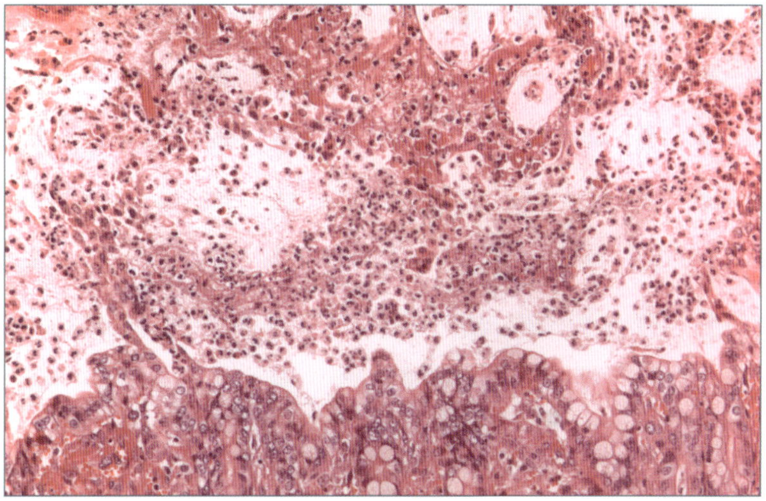

106B

106C **Fibrinous enteritis.** Fibrillar acidophilic material including neutrophils and erythrocytes in the intestinal submucosa. HE.

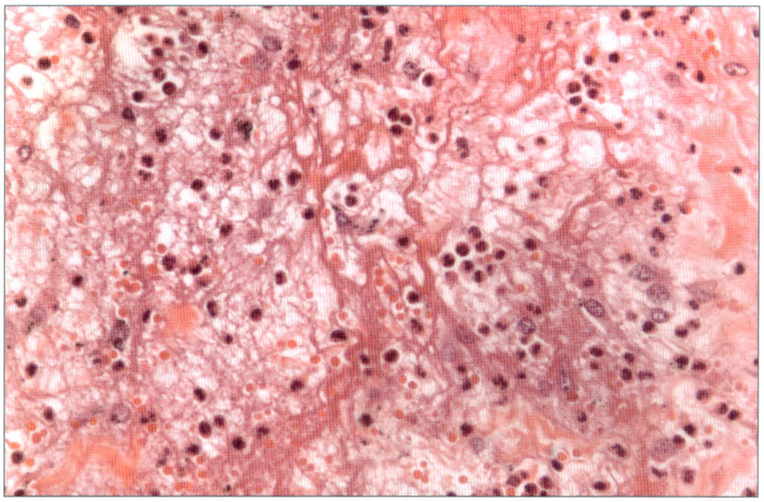

106C

107

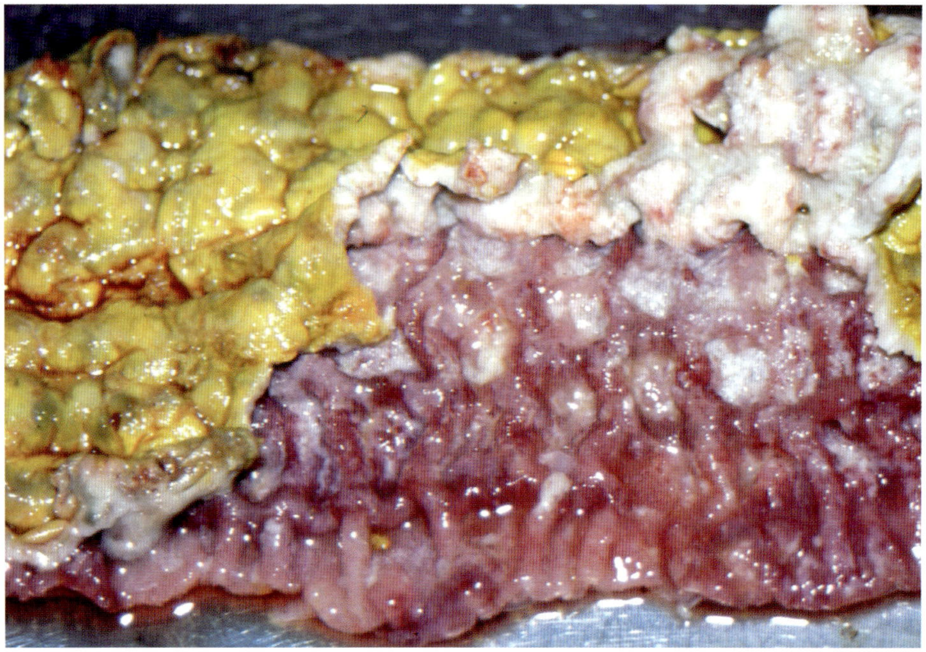

108A

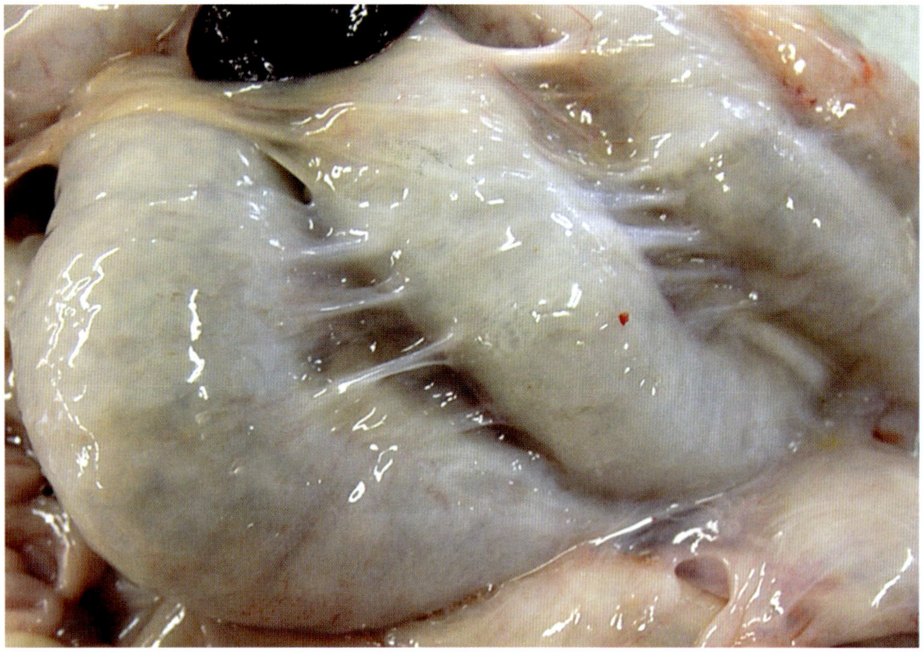

107 **Fibrinous exudate.**
Wrinkled, whitish pseudomembrane, with a yellow-stained outer surface, on a reddened ileal mucosa.

108A **Fibrinous colitis.**
Turgid large intestine: the serosa has a gelatinous aspect and the intestinal loops are separated by oedema. Weaner pig.

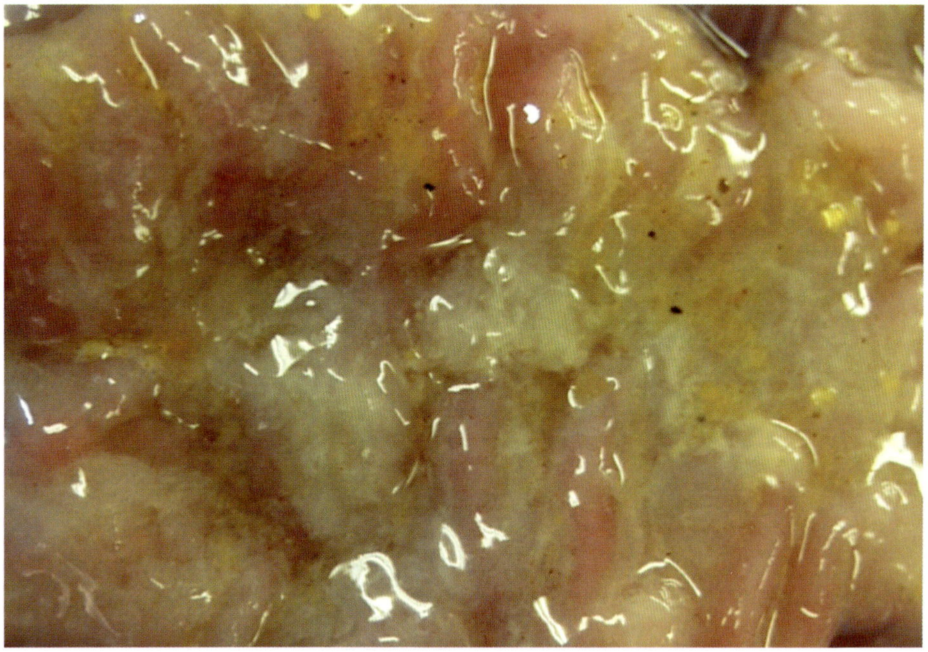

108B

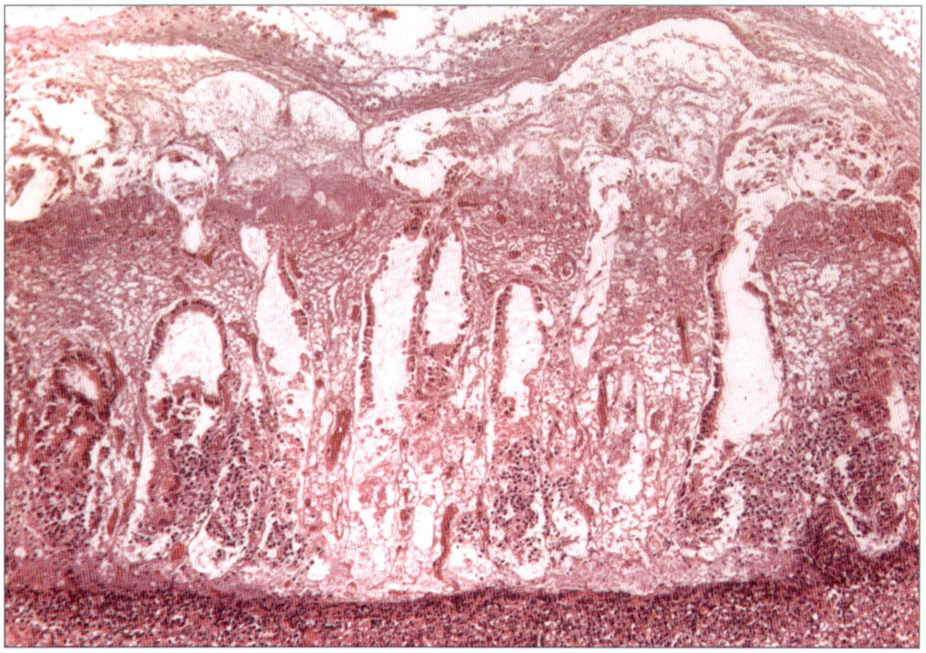

108C

108B Fibrinous colitis.
Thickened mucosa of the large intestine, with red foci and greyish deposits with a mucoid appearance. Weaner pig.

108C Fibrinous colitis.
Necrotic focus on the mucosa with some conservation of tissue layers, limited in depth by inflammatory cellular infiltrate and on the surface by an adherent pseudomembrane. HE.

109A

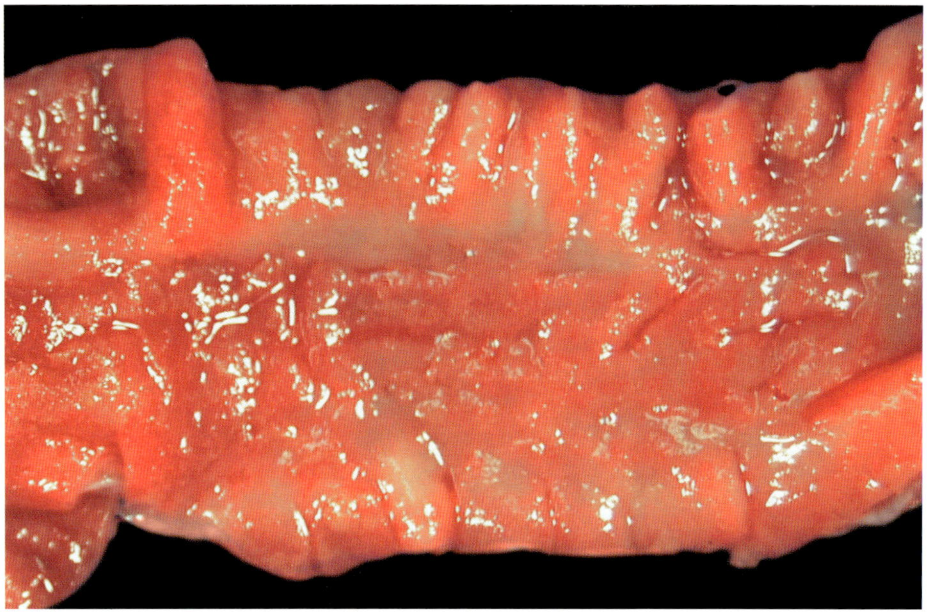

109B

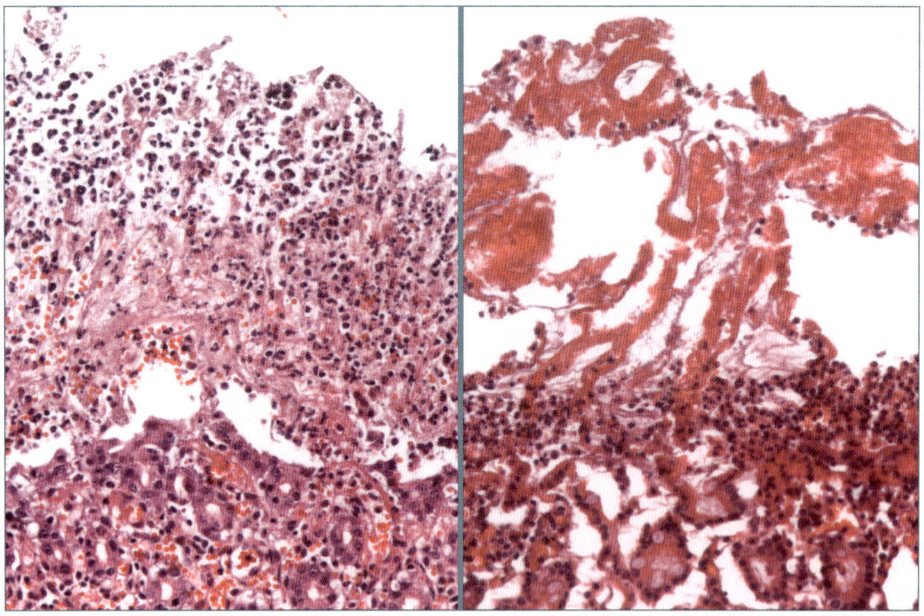

109A Fibrinous colitis.

The mucosa of the colon is thickened, reddened, and dotted with yellowish lumps and plaques. Weaner pig.

109B Fibrinous colitis.

Exudate consisting of fibrillar acidophilic material with cellular debris and inflammatory cells, anchored at certain points to the eroded mucosa (left). Pseudomembrane adhered to the altered intestinal mucosa in another segment (right). HE.

110A

Fibrinous colitis.

Segment of the colon with greyish, firmly adhered plaques arranged transversely on a dark red mucosa (left). Segment of colon with grey, irregular, coalescing plaques on a reddened and granular mucosal surface (right). Fattening pig.

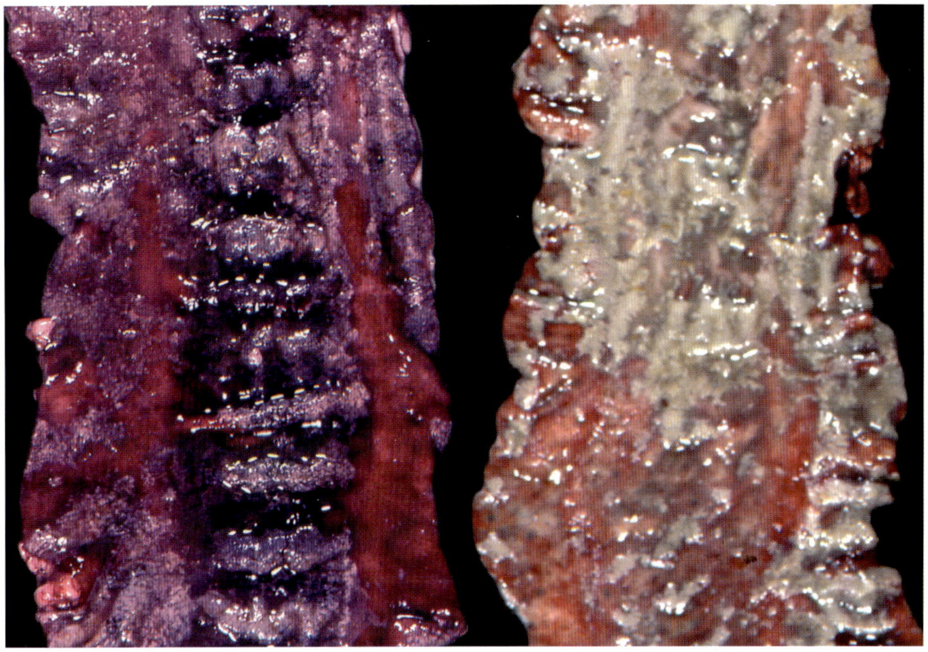

110A

110B

Fibrinous colitis.

Pseudomembranous exudate formed by the accumulation of fibrin, leukocytes, and epithelial cells with superficial mucosal necrosis. HE.

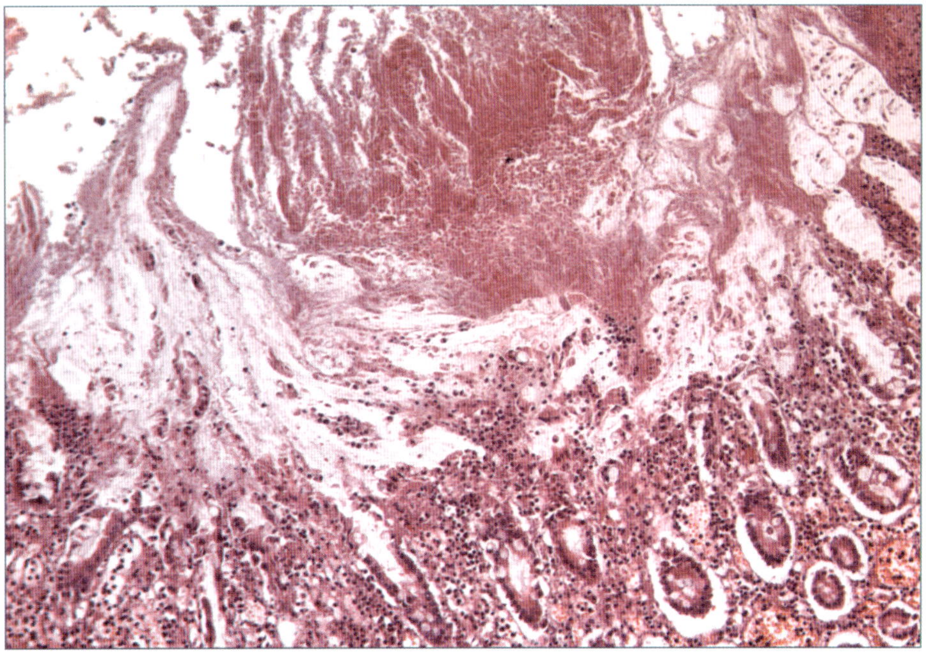

110B

Fibrinous enterocolitis is associated with salmonellosis and can be fibrinohaemorrhagic in postweaning colibacillosis. Diphtheritic typhlocolitis appears in dysentery (generally in the fibrinohaemorrhagic form), salmonellosis, trichuriasis, and in some severe cases of spirochetosis. Salmonellosis and classical swine fever present with diphtheroid lesions of the lymphoid follicles of the colon.

Necrotic inflammation

111A

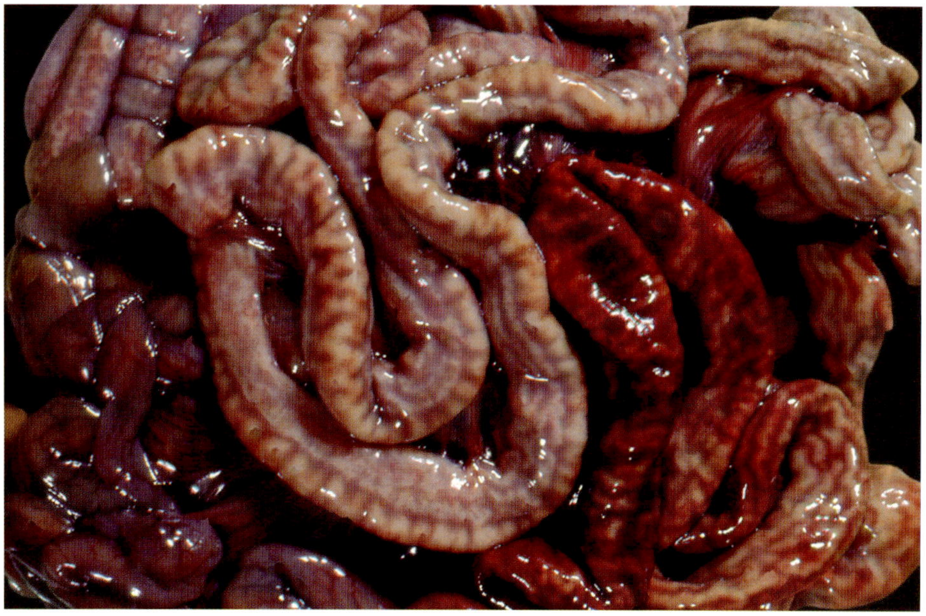

111B

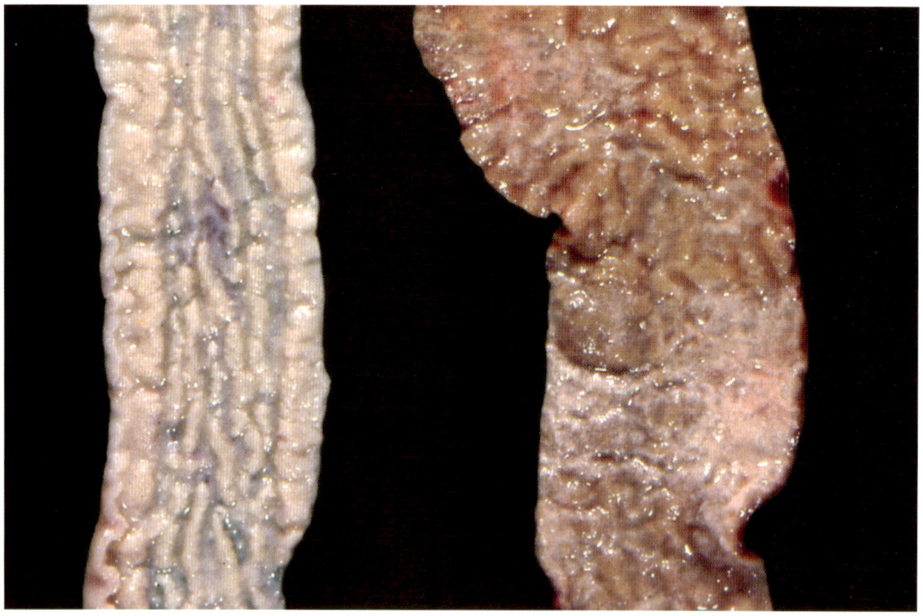

111A Necrotic enteritis.
Turgid loops of the small intestine: some segments have a reticulated appearance, while others display a marbled red colouring. Suckling pig.

111B Necrotic enteritis.
Segments of the small intestine with rough whitish mucosa and foci of red discolouration.

112A Necrotic enteritis.

Loops of the small intestine displaying intense red discolouration, with subserosal bubbles produced by parietal emphysema. Suckling pig.

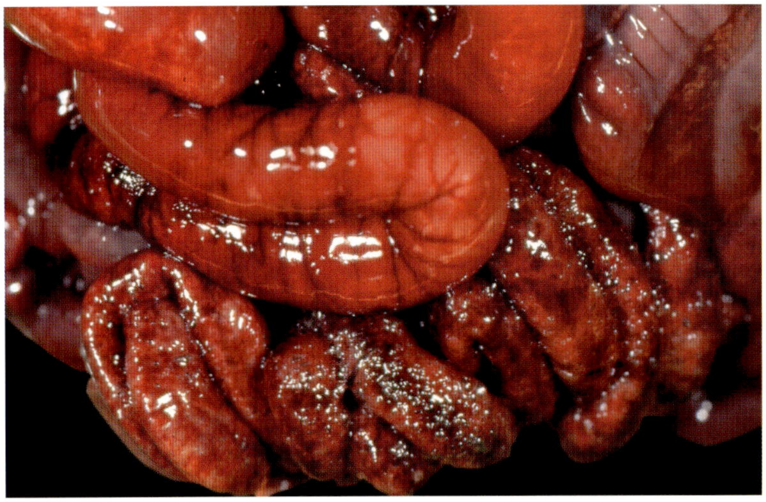
112A

112B Necrotic enteritis.

Wrinkled, whitish mucosa of the small intestine showing mild reddish discolouration.

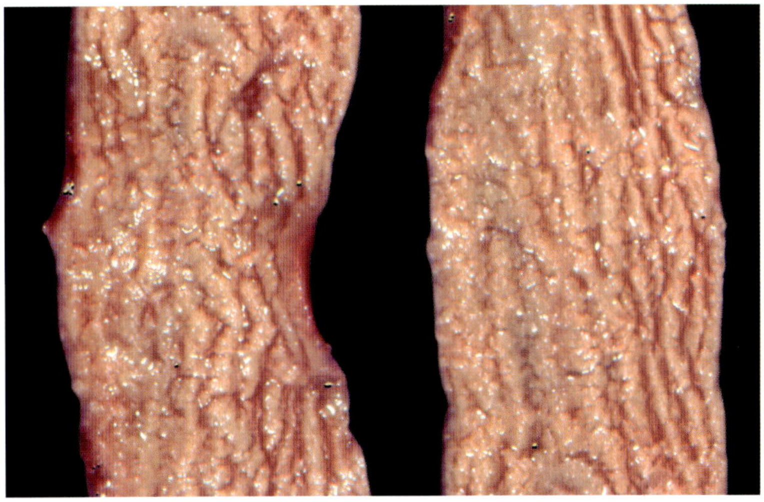
112B

112C Necrotic enteritis.

Mucosal necrosis with inflammatory infiltration, parietal haemorrhage, and intramural emphysema, as evidenced by the presence of optically empty spaces. HE.

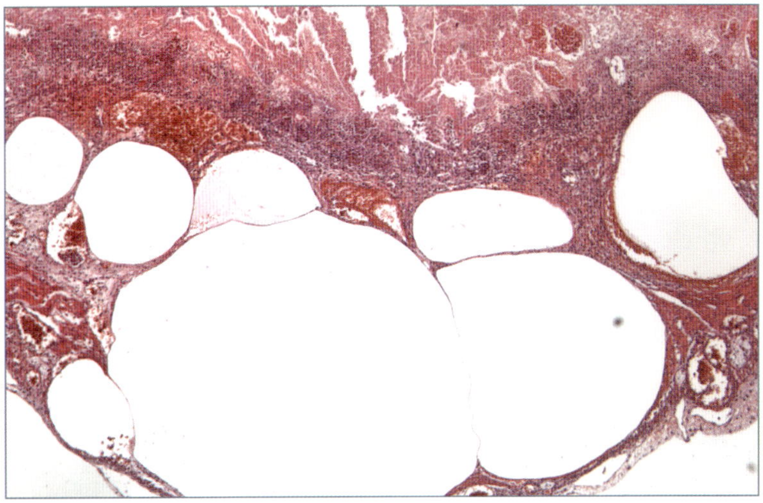
112C

113A

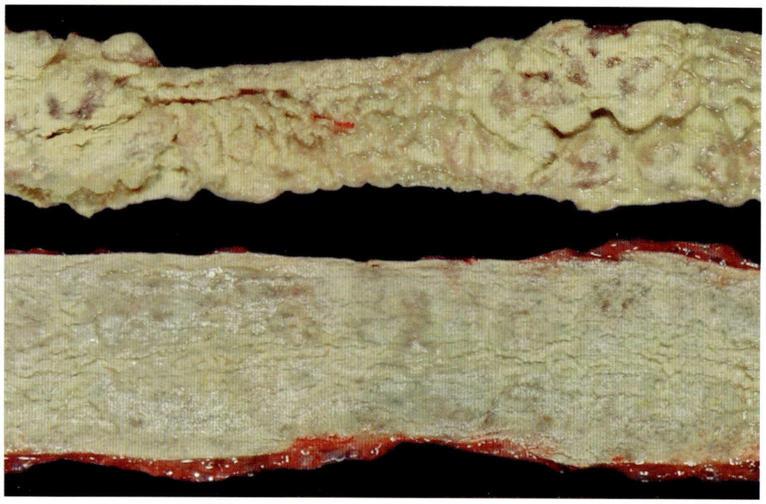

113A **Necrotic enteritis.**
Segments of the small intestine with dull, whitish, rough and fissured mucosa. Suckling pig.

113B

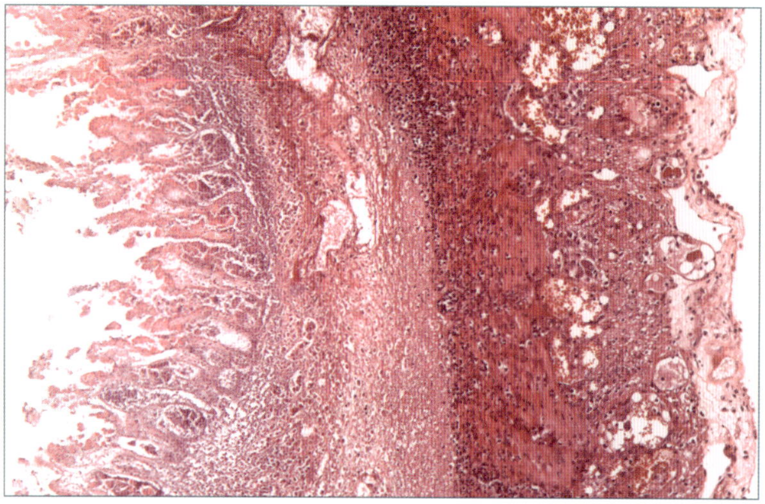

113B **Necrotic enteritis.**
Alteration of the mucosa showing remnants of villi, hyperaemia, and intraparietal haemorrhage. HE.

113C

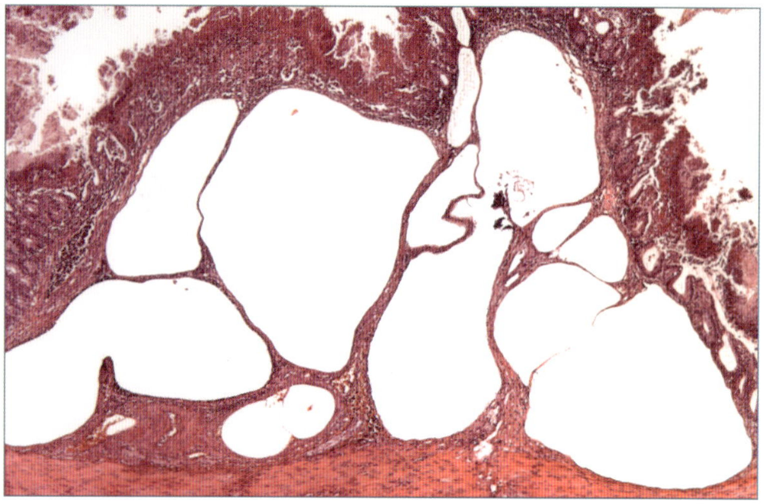

113C **Necrotic enteritis.**
Intestinal wall showing extensive necrosis of the mucosa and large optically empty spaces that cause dilation of the submucosa, corresponding to emphysema. HE.

114A

Necrotic enteritis. Segments of small intestine, some reddened and others showing clear longitudinal lines that are visible through the serosa. Suckling pig.

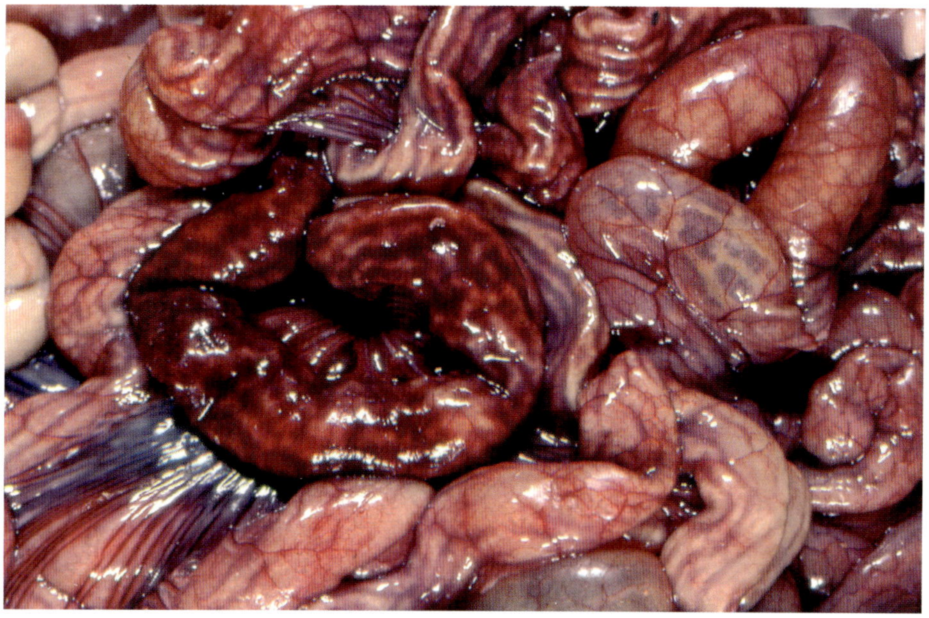

114A

114B

Necrotic enteritis. Destruction of the mucosa with preservation of tissue contours and underlying inflammatory demarcation. HE.

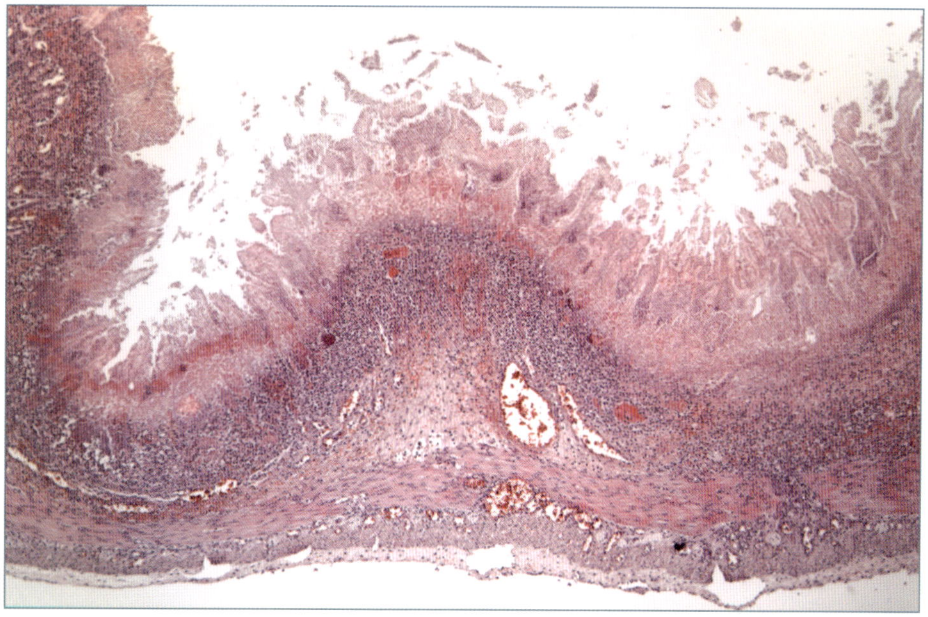

114B

Lesions caused by necrotic enteritis due to *C. perfringens* type C in piglets affect the small intestine, and in some cases the proximal portion of the large intestine. One form of superficial necrotising enterocolitis is associated with *C. perfringens* type A infection in lactating animals. These alterations may also appear in haemorrhagic *E. coli* gastroenteritis.

115A

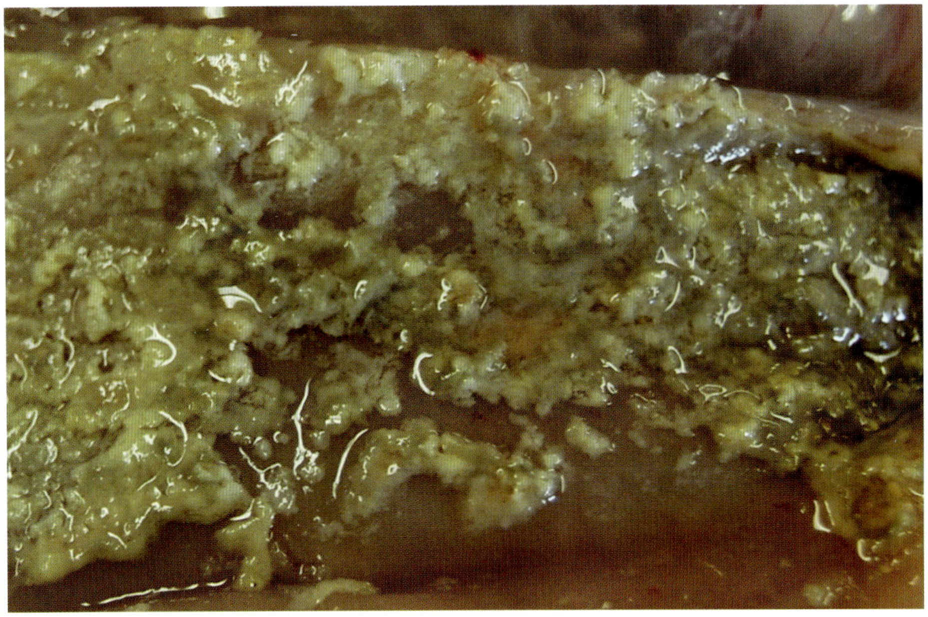

115B

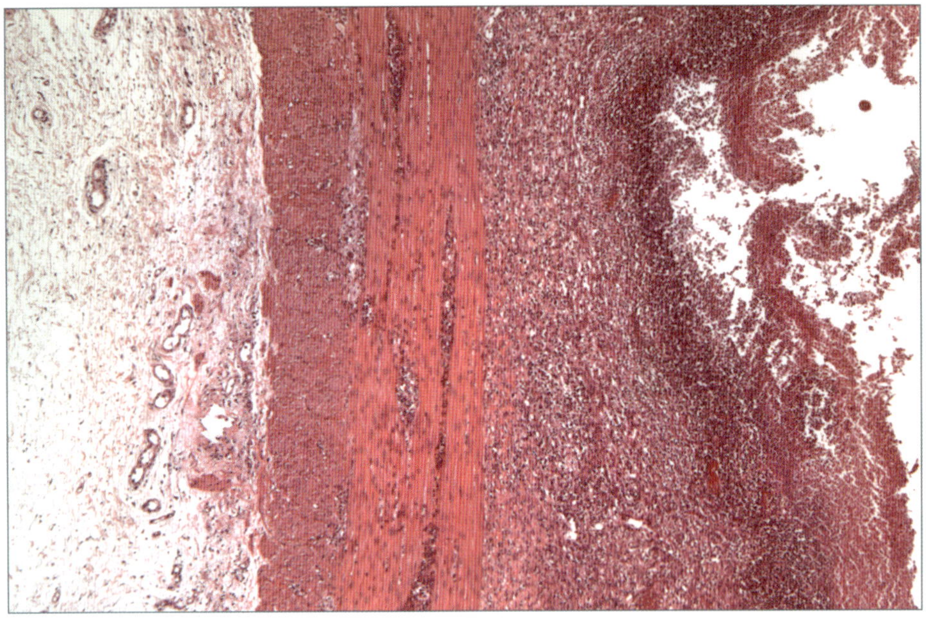

115A Necrotic colitis.
Furfuraceous colonic mucosa on which foci of erosion with a smooth base can be observed. Weaner pig.

115B Necrotic colitis.
Focus of tissue destruction, which is demarcated by the inflammatory reaction, affecting the partially detached mucosa. HE.

116A Necrotic colitis.

Loops of the colon with foci that are visible through the serosa due to the irregular thickness of the intestinal wall. Weaner pig.

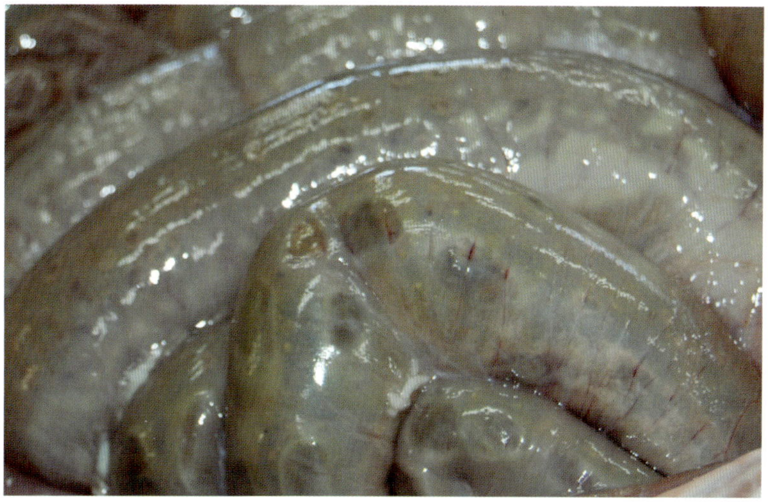

116A

116B Necrotic colitis.

Greyish confluent plaques adhering to the mucosa of the large intestine. Weaner pig.

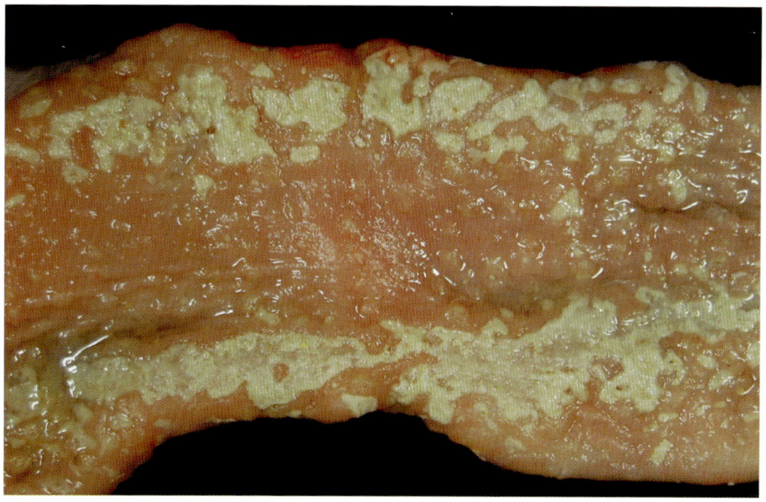

116B

116C Necrotic colitis.

Focus of mucosal alteration demarcated by inflammatory infiltrate and limited marginally by normal mucosa. HE.

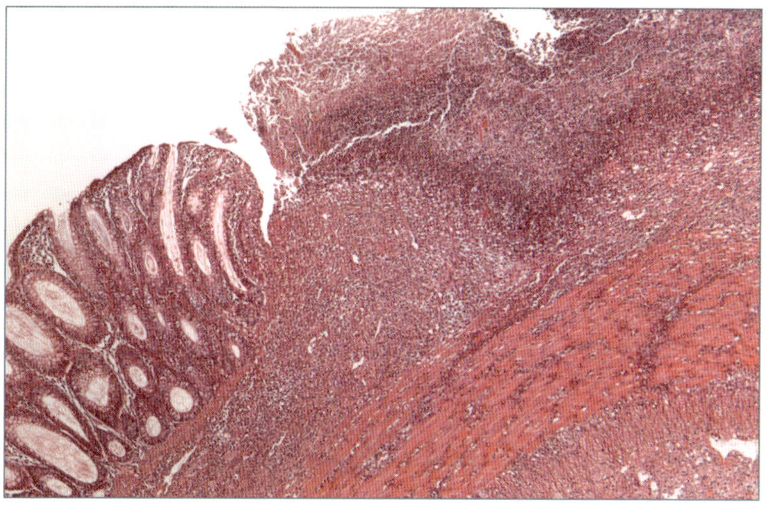

116C

117A

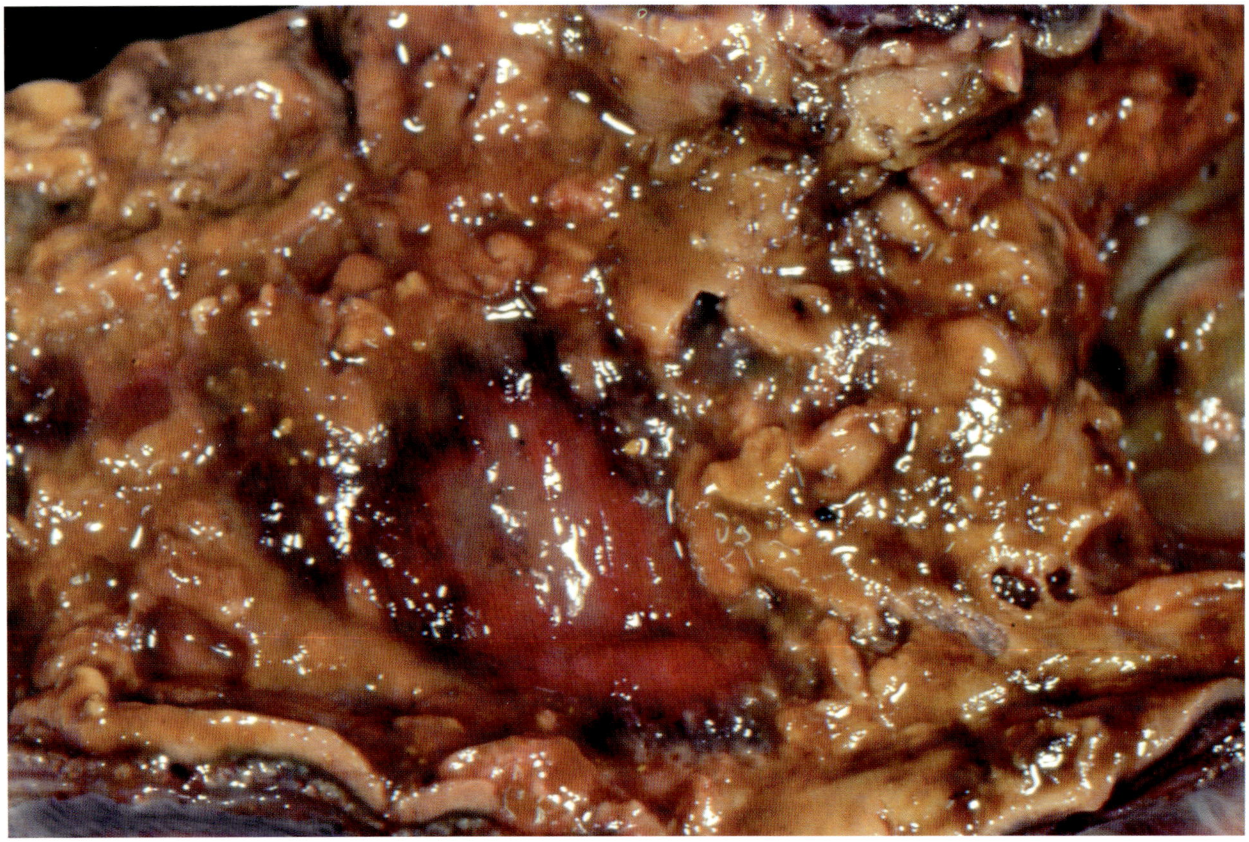

117A Necrotic colitis.
Yellowish anfractuous mucosa of the large intestine that has detached in one area, leaving a red focus. Fattening pig.

117B

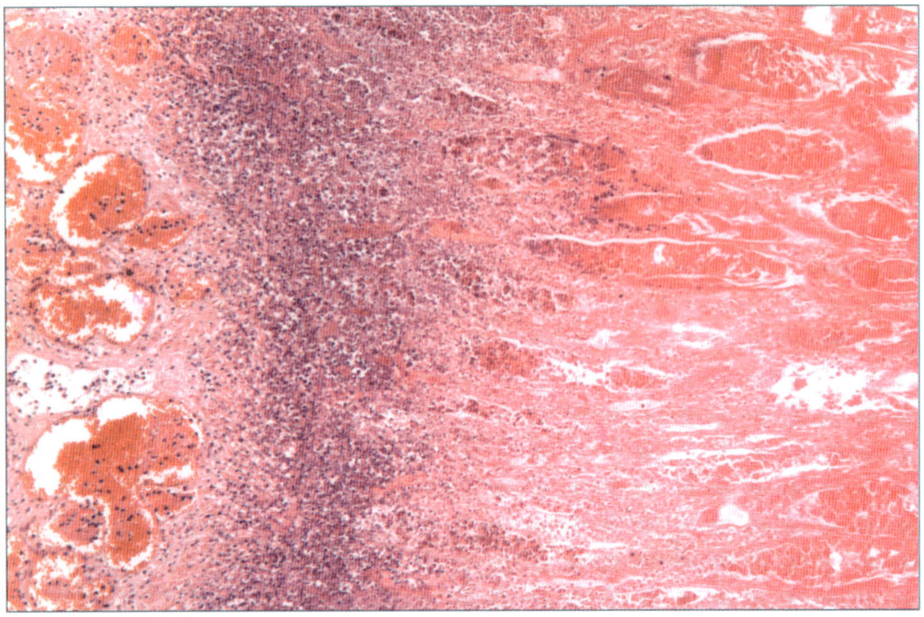

117B
Necrotic colitis.
Mucosal necrosis defined by diffuse eosinophilia and relative conservation of tissue layers, separated from the submucosa by a band of cellular debris, leukocytes, and bacterial colonies. HE.

118A

Necrotic colitis.

Mild, greyish to black foci of excavation in the reddened and thickened mucosa of the colon. Fattening pig.

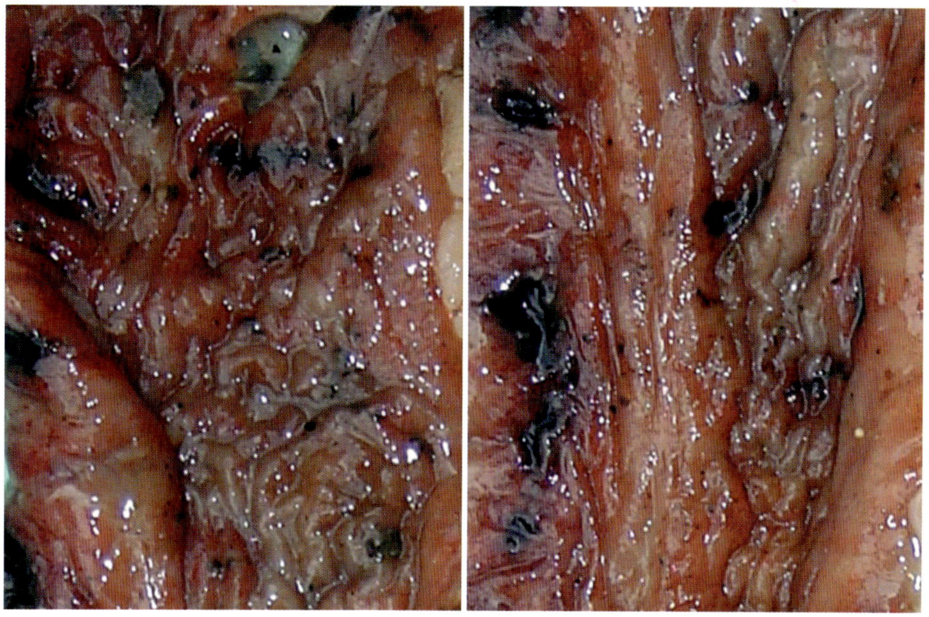

118A

118B

Necrotic colitis.

Necrosis of the mucosa, with partial conservation of structure and pronounced inflammatory demarcation. HE.

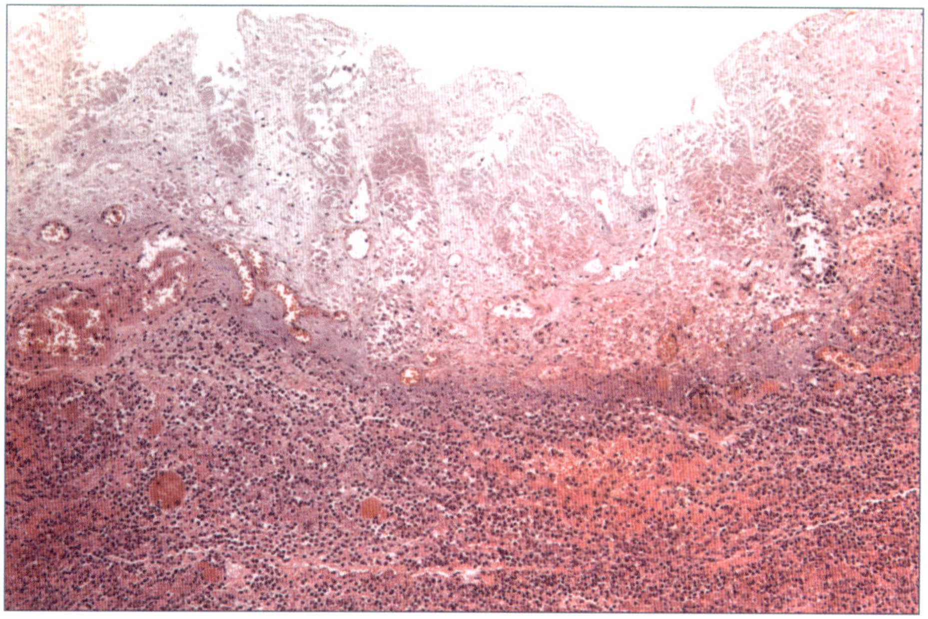

118B

Deep, focal, and diffuse necrotic typhlocolitis has been linked to salmonellosis. In the enterocolitic form the ileal necrosis is usually superficial. It has been suggested that porcine circovirus is a causative agent of necrotising enterocolitis.

Proliferative enteropathy

The associated microscopic lesions are characterised by the proliferation of immature epithelial crypt cells. The inflammatory reaction is not a primary characteristic, and depends on the evolution of the process. Porcine proliferative enteropathy groups together the morphopathological variants previously included in the so-called intestinal adenomatosis complex.

119A

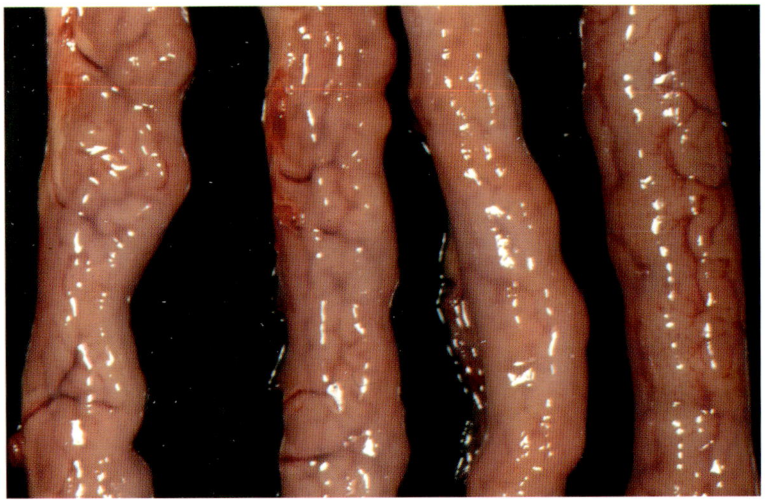

119A Proliferative enteropathy. The affected segments of the small intestine are pale and turgid, with an irregular profile. Fattening pig.

119B

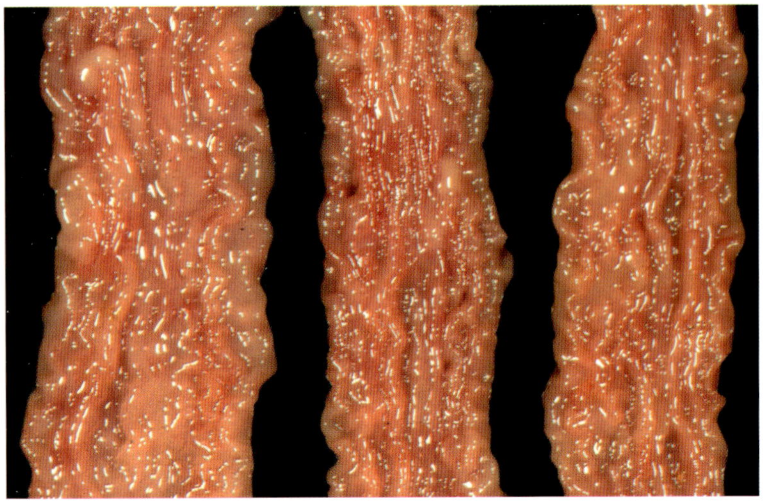

119B Proliferative enteropathy. Thickened mucosa of the small intestine with foci of nodules or pseudopolyp-like lesions. Fattening pig.

120 **Proliferative enteropathy.** Epithelial hyperplasia of the crypts of the small intestine with leukocytes and cellular debris in the lumina. Fattening pig. HE.

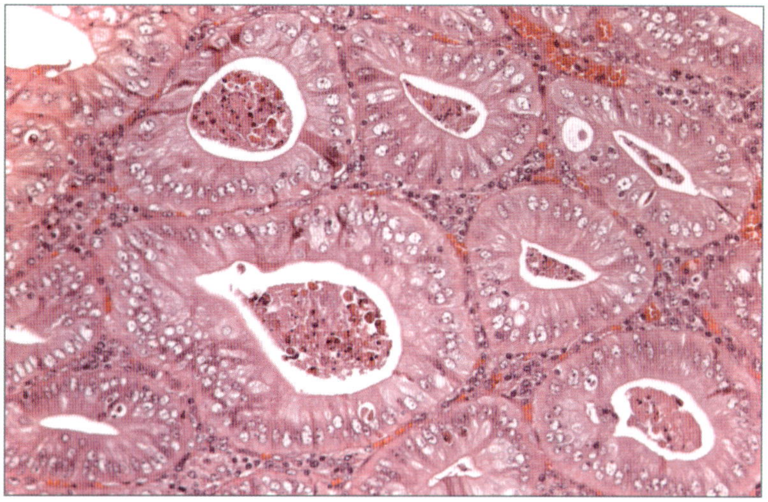

120

121 **Proliferative enteropathy.** Epithelial proliferation of the crypts of the large intestine, with inflammatory cells and cellular debris in the lumina. Lamina propria infiltrated by inflammatory cells. HE.

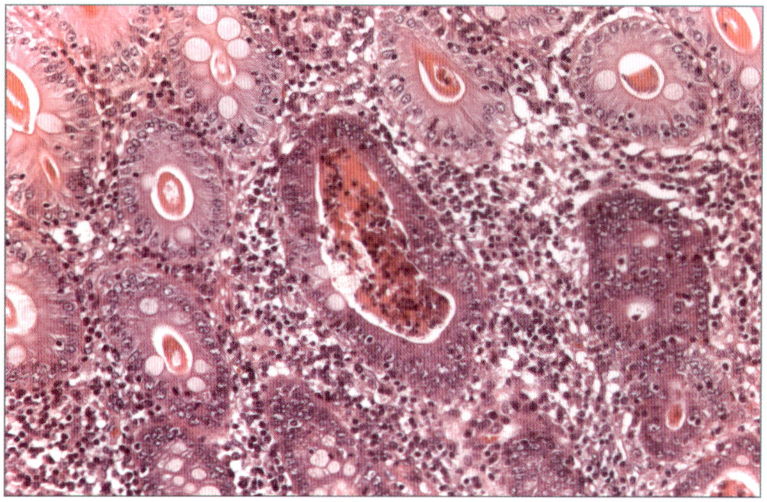

121

122 **Proliferative enteropathy.** Diphtheroid, tubular pseudomembrane detatched from the surface of the small intestine. In some areas the prominent relief of the hyperplastic mucosa is adopted by the luminal surface. Complicated form of proliferative enteropathy. Fattening pig. HE.

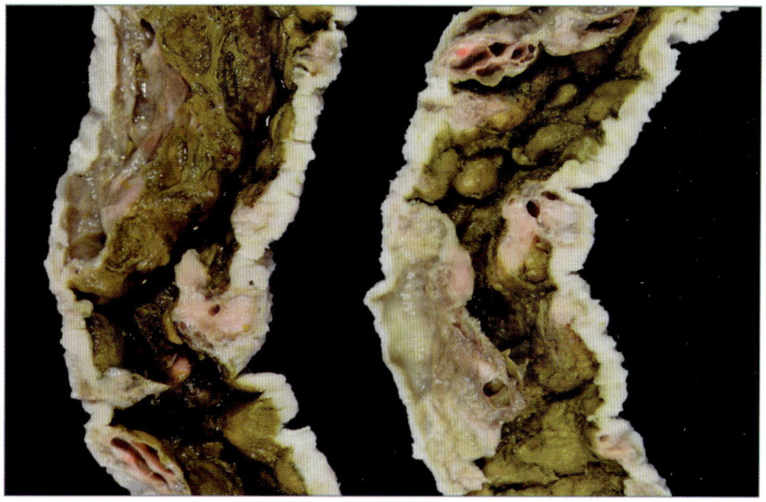

122

123A

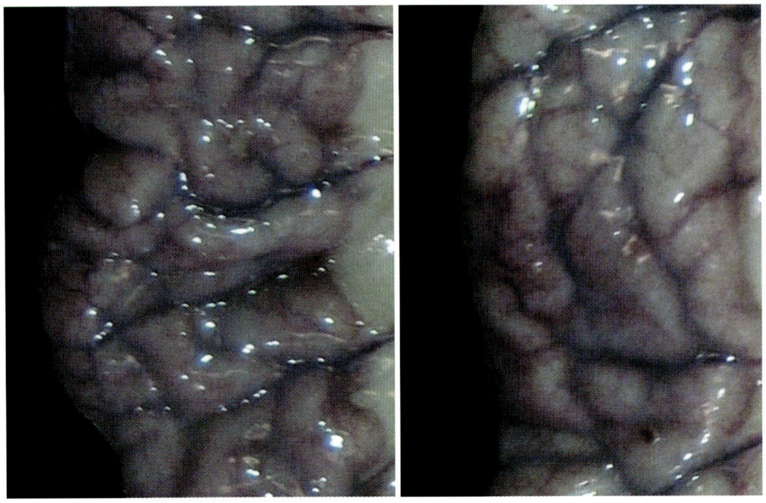

123A **Proliferative enteropathy.** Reticulated serosa of the small intestine, imitating the pattern of cerebral gyri. Fattening pig.

123B

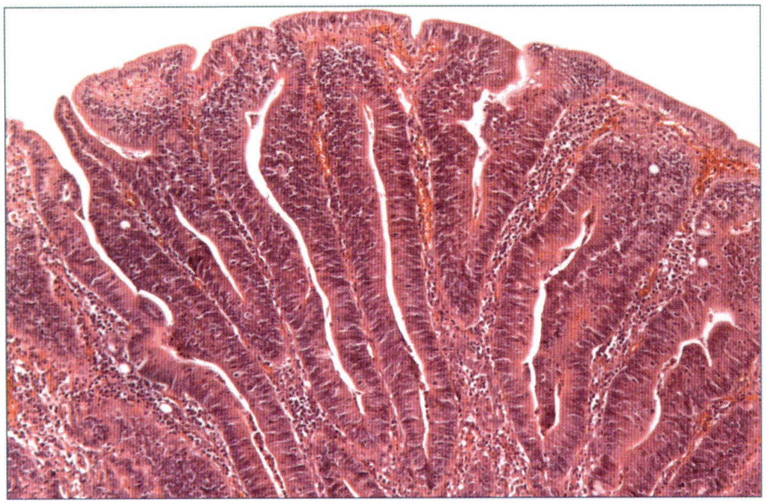

123B **Proliferative enteropathy.** Expansion and lengthening of the intestinal crypts, which extend to the surface of a flattened mucosa, with loss of goblet cells. HE.

123C

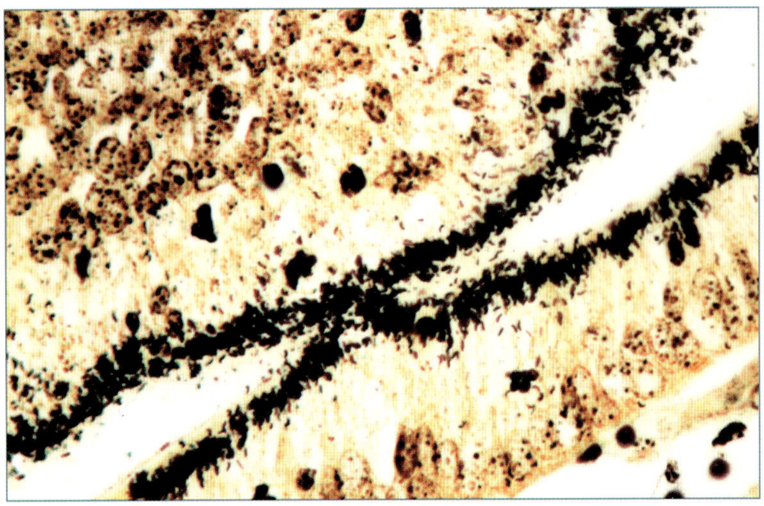

123C **Proliferative enteropathy.** Dense line of black-stained bacteria in the apical cytoplasm of the proliferating enterocytes of an intestinal crypt. WS.

124A **Proliferative enteropathy.** Cerebriform serosa of the small intestine (left). Marked mucosal folds (right). Fattening pig.

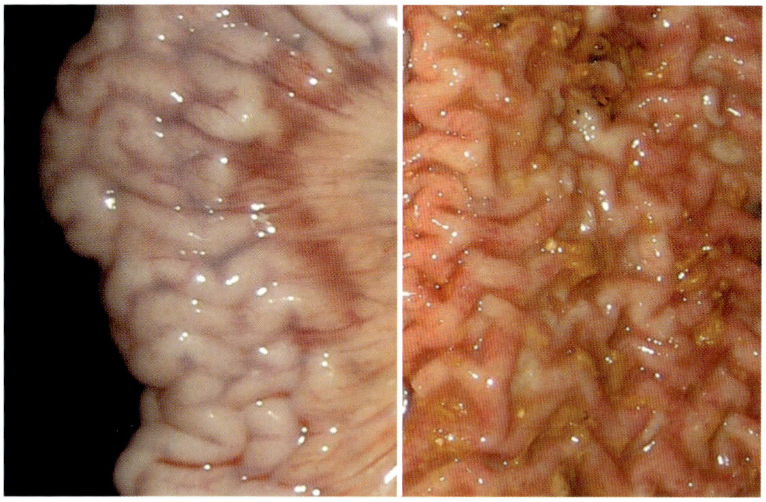

124A

124B **Proliferative enteropathy.** Marked increase in the epithelial cells of the crypts, some of which contain inflammatory cells and cellular debris in their dilated lumina. HE.

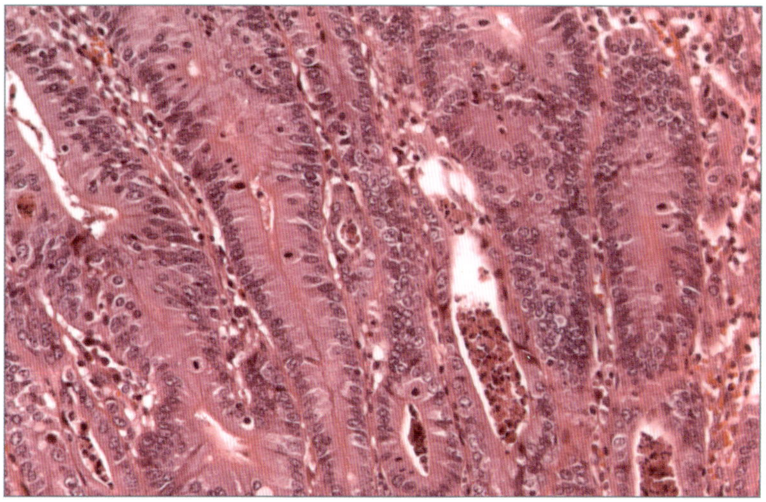

124B

125A **Proliferative enteropathy.** Turgid, pale loops of the small intestine exhibiting an irregular profile. Fattening pig.

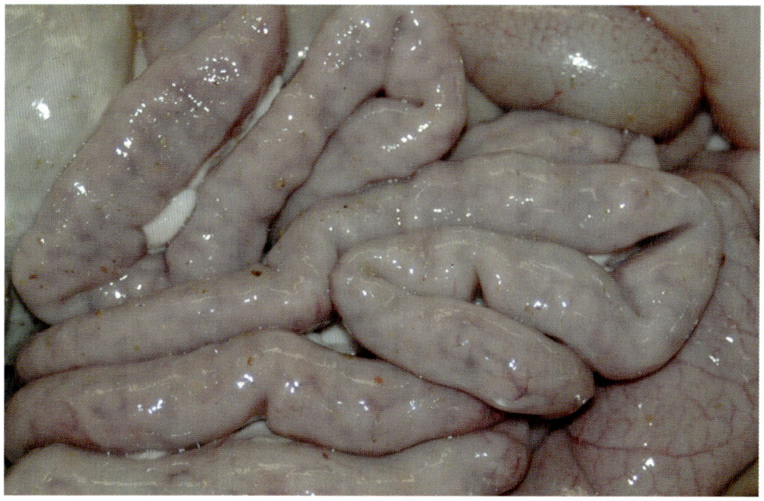

125A

125B

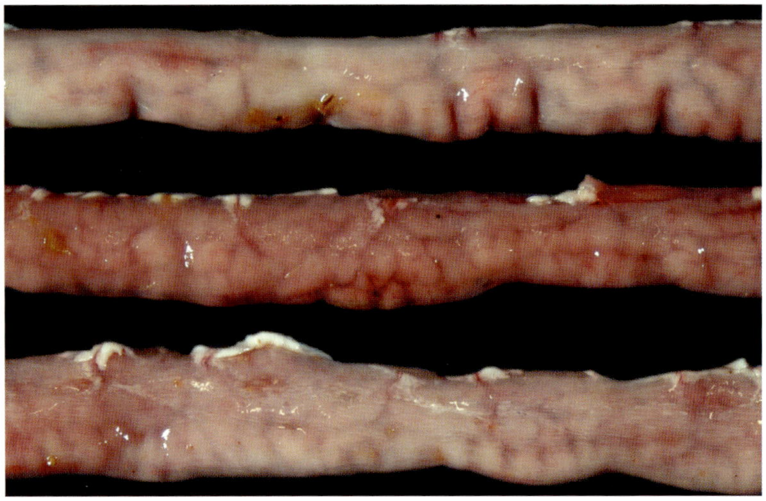

125B Proliferative enteropathy.
Segments of the small intestine displaying a dentate appearance with reticulated serosa.

125C

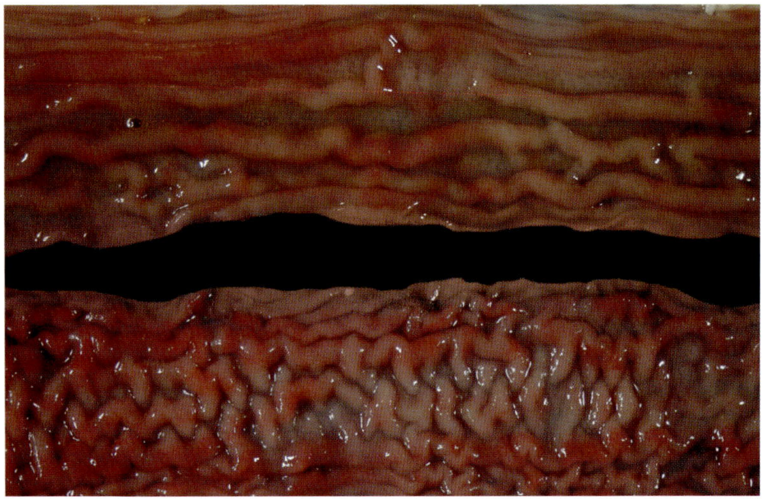

125C Proliferative enteropathy.
Thickening of the mucosal folds of the small intestine in a linear or cerebriform pattern, depending on the evolution of the process in the affected segments.

125D

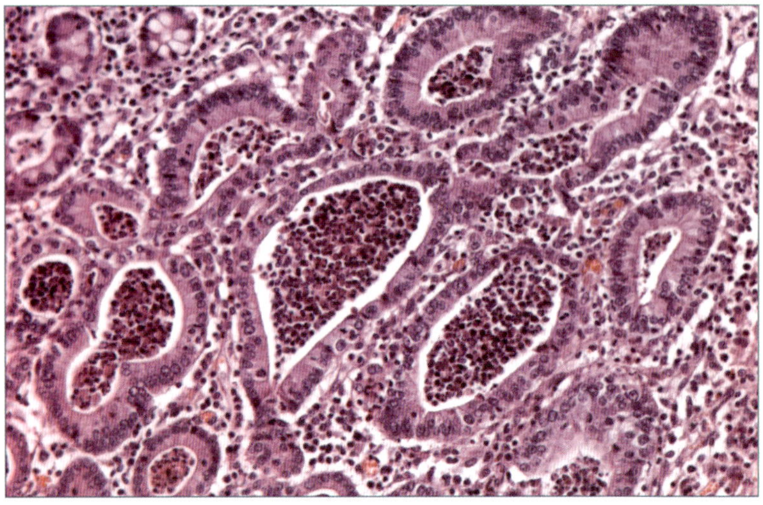

125D Proliferative enteropathy.
Hyperplastic crypts, devoid of goblet cells, with cellular debris and inflammatory cells in the dilated lumina. Lamina propria infiltrated by inflammatory cells. HE.

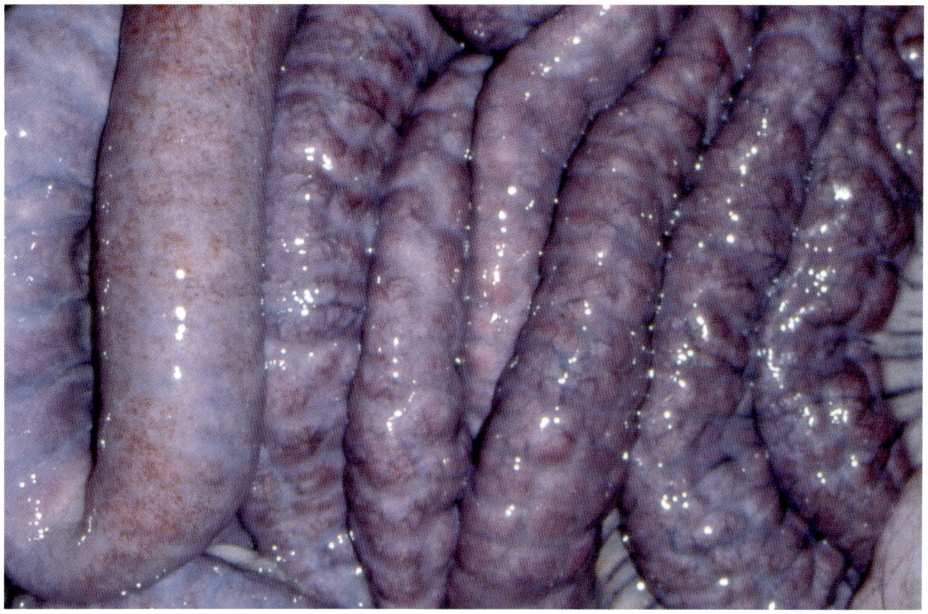

126A

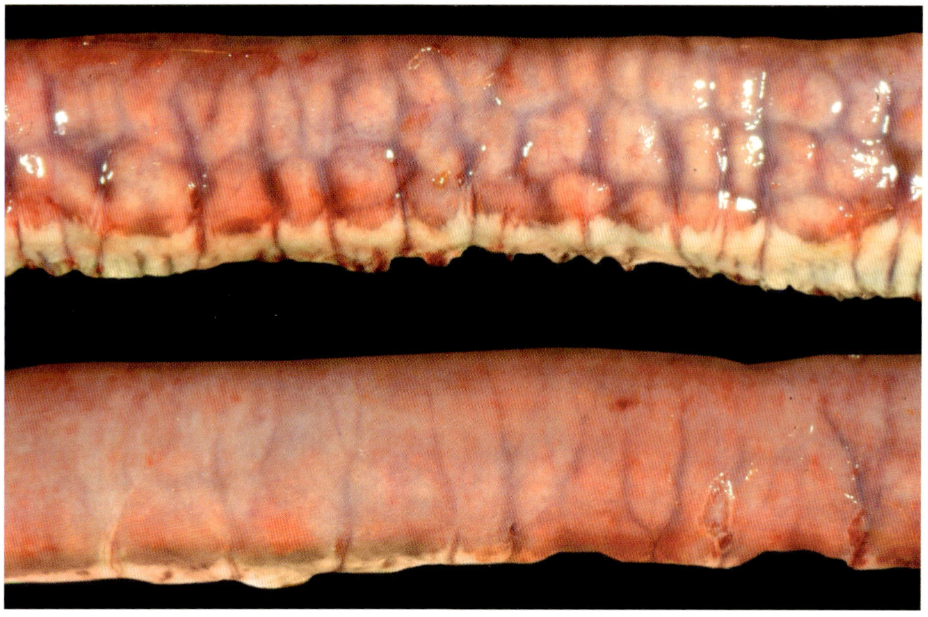

126B

126A Proliferative enteropathy.
Thickened, turgid segments of the small intestine displaying increased colouration and an irregular serosal surface. Replacement sow.

126B Proliferative enteropathy.
Thickened and swollen segments of the small intestine. The reticular pattern of the serosa is more pronounced in one segment (cobblestone-like appearance).

126C

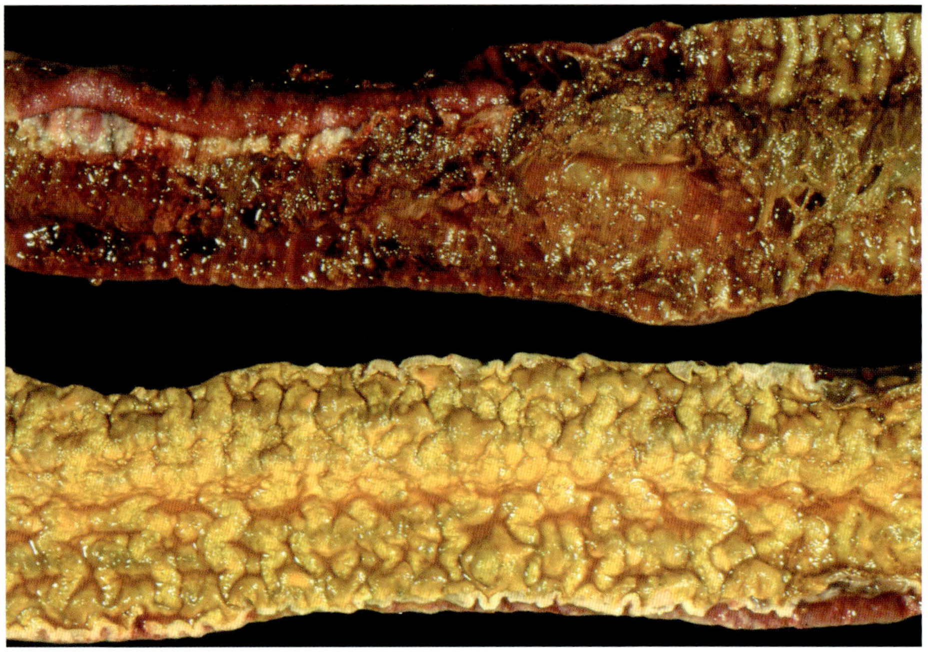

126D

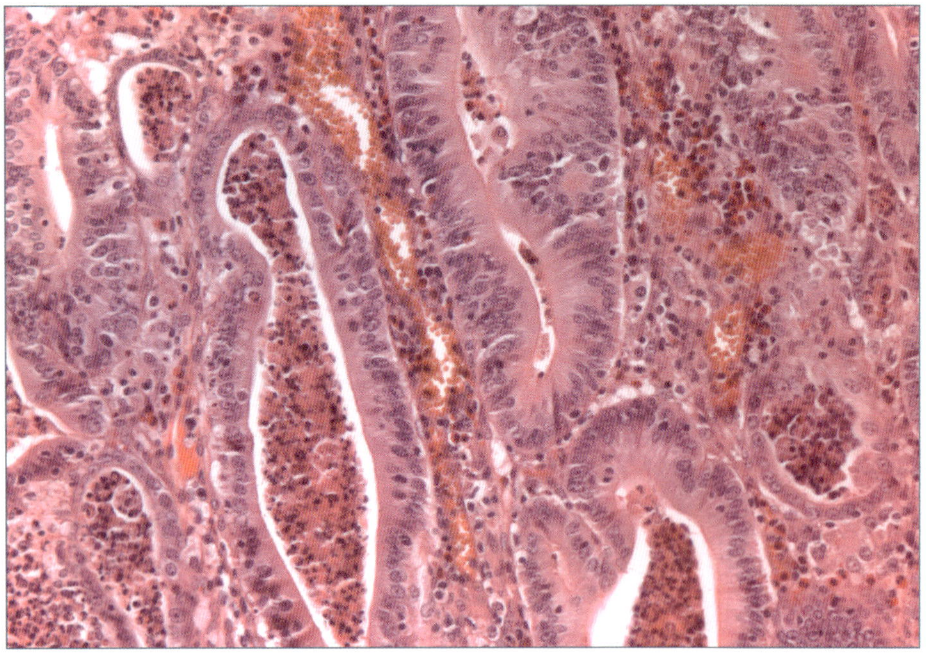

126C Proliferative enteropathy.
Anfractuous mucosa of the small intestine, with brownish discolouration, reddish foci, and mucosal detachment in some areas (top). Yellowish pseudomembrane which adopts the shape of the proliferative mucosa of the small intestine (bottom).

126D Proliferative enteropathy.
Crypts exhibiting marked development due to hyperplasia of immature enterocytes, with accumulation of cellular and inflammatory debris in the lumina. HE.

126E

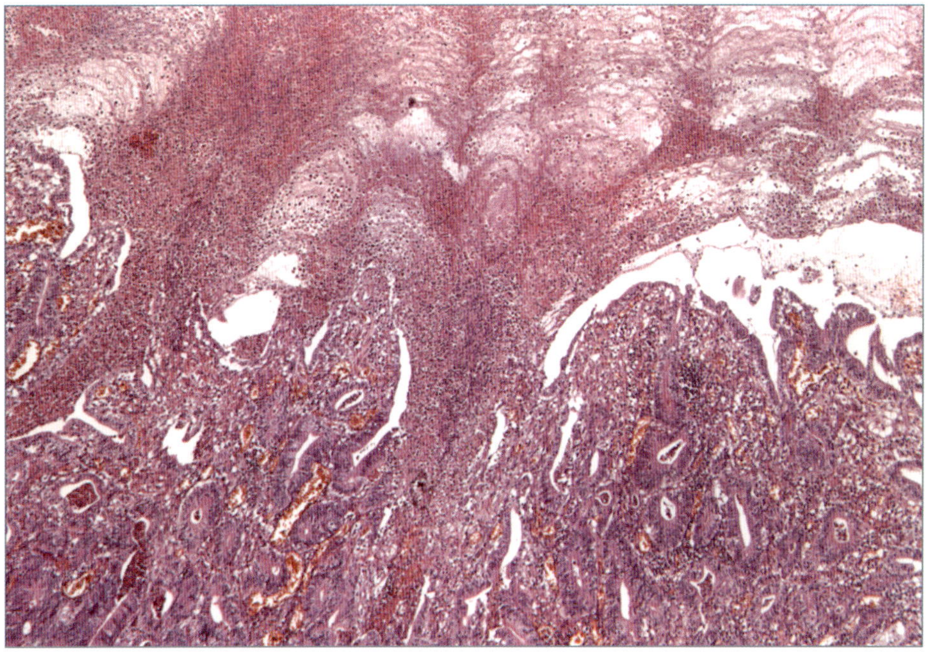

126E

Proliferative enteropathy. Pseudomembranous exudate displaying a laminar profile with focal alteration of the prolferative mucosa. HE.

126F

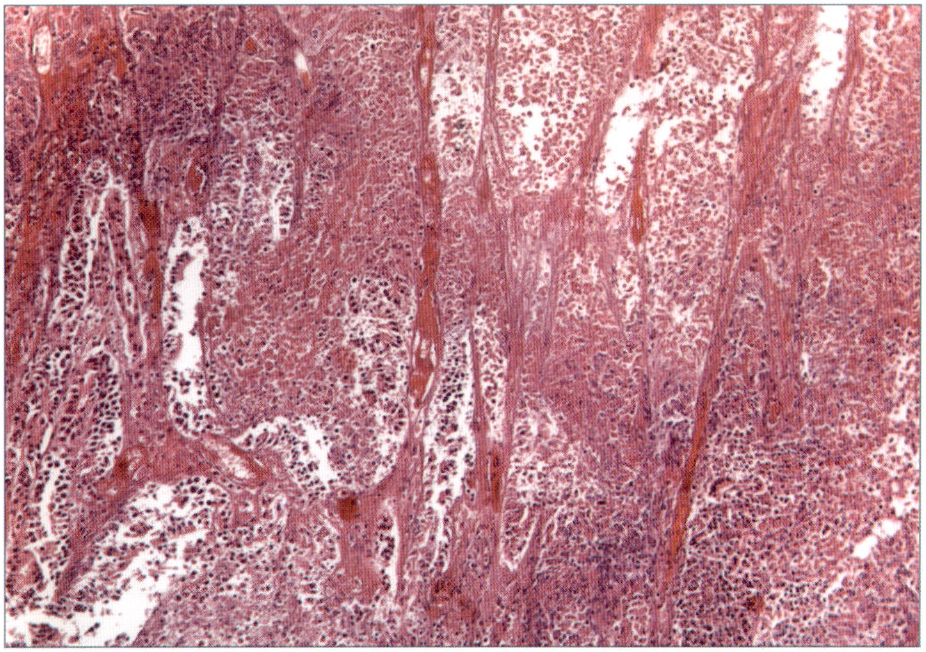

126F

Proliferative enteropathy. Coagulative necrosis superimposed upon a proliferative mucosal lesion. HE.

Lesions in proliferative enteropathy associated with *Lawsonia intracellularis* infection are located in the ileum, but may extend cranially and in some cases involve the proximal large intestine. Morphology is variable, depending on complications of the primary lesion.

Chronic nonproliferative inflammation

This is characterised by persistent cellular infiltrate without marked tissue neoformation. The morphology of some of these alterations, classified as chronic catarrhal inflammation, is similar to that of the entities described as lymphoplasmacytic enteritis and idiopathic colitis in other species.

127A

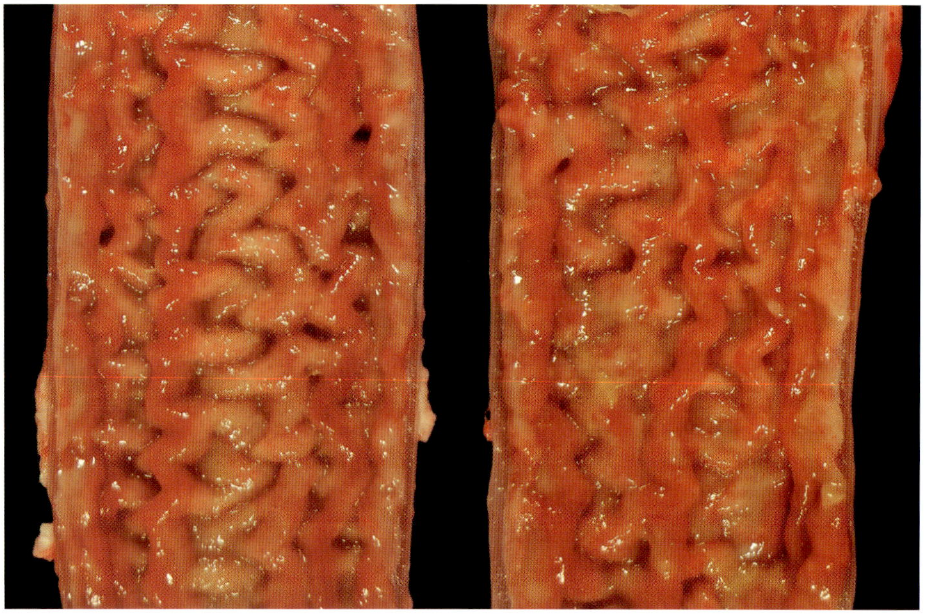

127B

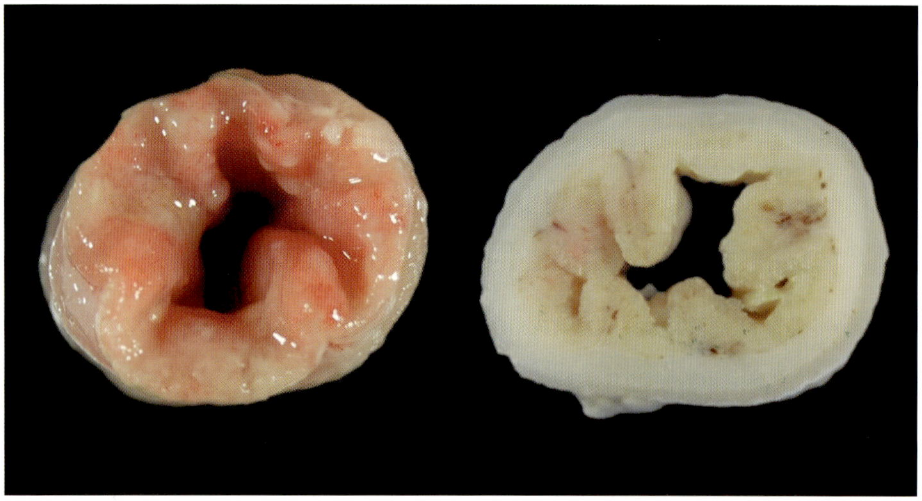

127A Chronic nonproliferative enteritis. Accentuated folds in the mucosa of the small intestine. Fattening pig.

127B Chronic nonproliferative enteritis. Thickening of the mucosa of the small intestine in a fresh sample (left) and in a fixed sample (right).

127C **Chronic nonproliferative enteritis.**
Expansion of the lamina propria caused by a dense lymphoplasmacytic and eosinophilic infiltrate. Elongated crypts, with numerous goblet cells. HE.

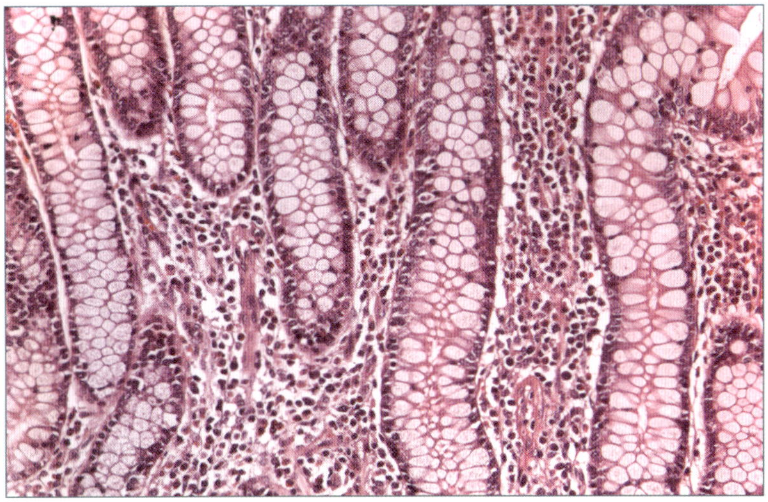
127C

128A **Chronic nonproliferative enteritis.**
Turgid loops of the small intestine, with irregular profile and loss of colour. Fattening pig.

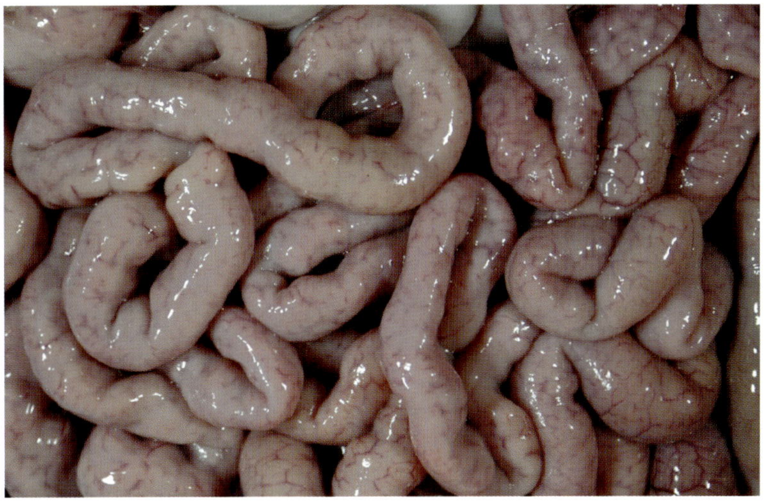
128A

128B **Chronic nonproliferative enteritis.**
Lamina propria dilated by the presence of a predominantly lymphoplasmacytic inflammatory cell infiltrate (left) and neutrophils in the lumina of some crypts (right). HE.

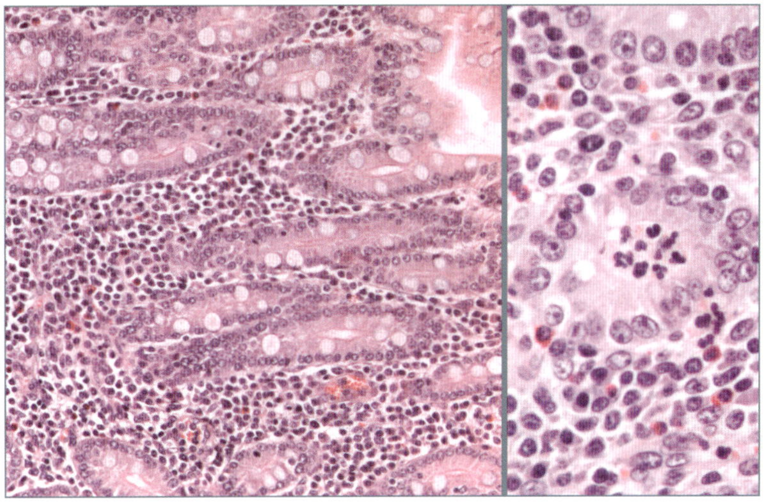
128B

129A

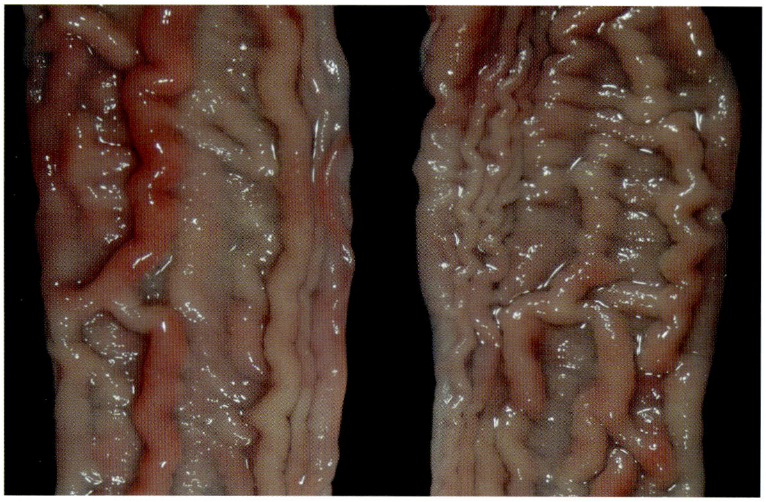

129A Chronic nonproliferative enteritis.

Thickening and focal reddening of the folds of the mucosa of the small intestine. Fattening pig.

129B

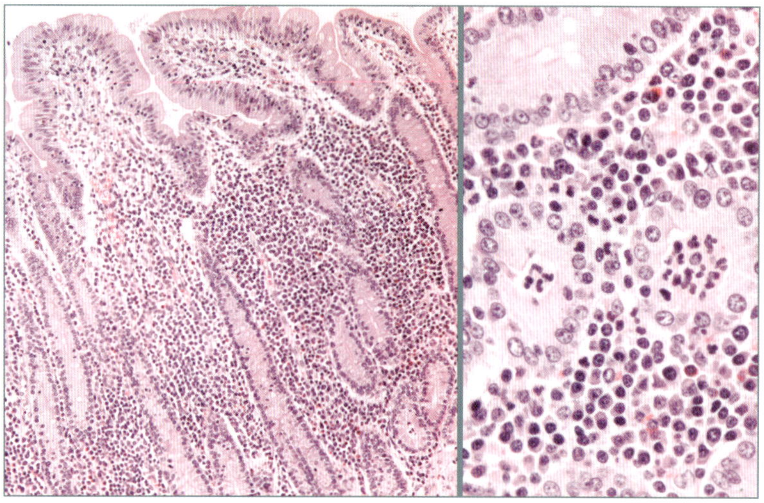

129B Chronic nonproliferative enteritis.

Enlargement of the lamina propria caused by inflammatory cell infiltrate (left). Predominantly lymphoplasmacytic inflammatory infiltrate in the lamina propria and crypt microabscesses (right). HE.

The main finding in nonproliferative enteritis is infiltration of the lamina propria with lymphocytes and plasma cells, with possible epithelial alterations and modification of the length of the villi. This finding is sometimes associated with systemic processes.

130A Chronic nonproliferative colitis.
Turgid large intestine. Suckling pig at end of lactation period.

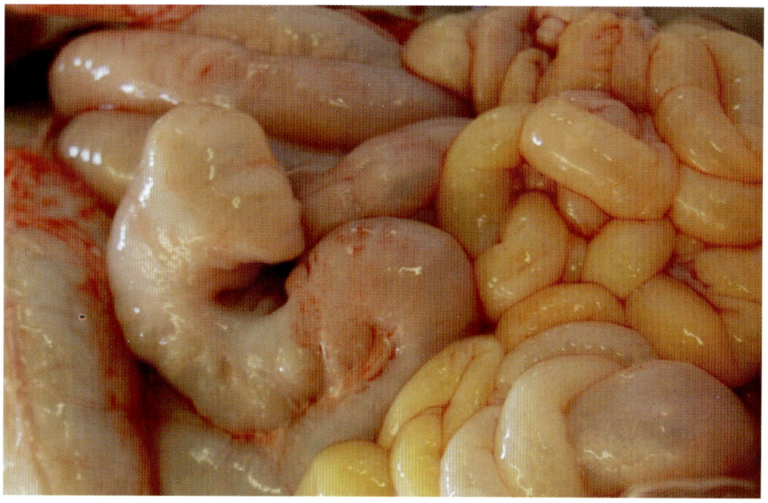
130A

130B Chronic nonproliferative colitis.
Inflammatory cell infiltrate in the lamina propria of the large intestine. HE.

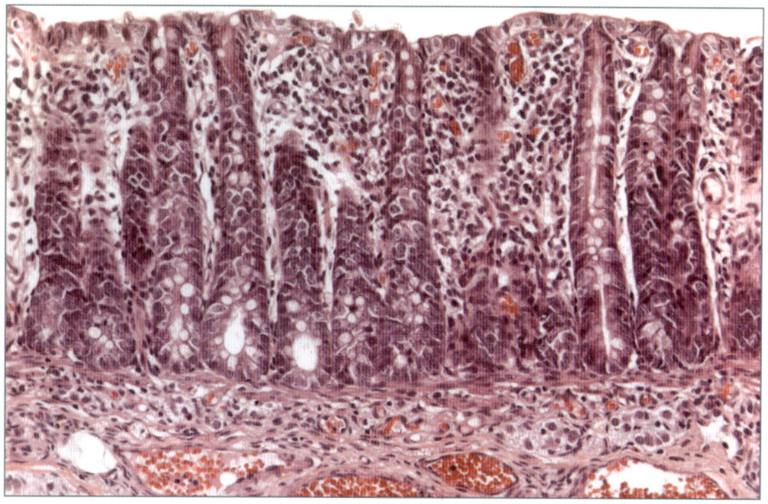
130B

130C Chronic nonproliferative colitis.
Crypts containing numerous black-stained spiral bacteria (left). Large numbers of spiral bacteria on the mucosal surface (right). WS.

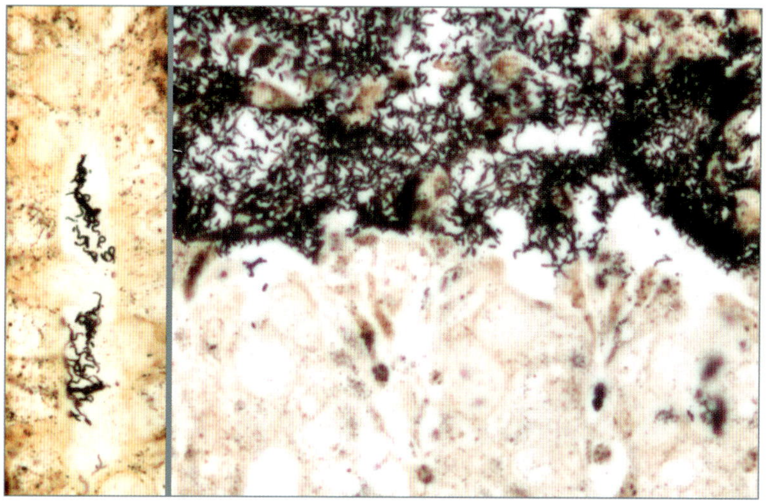
130C

131A

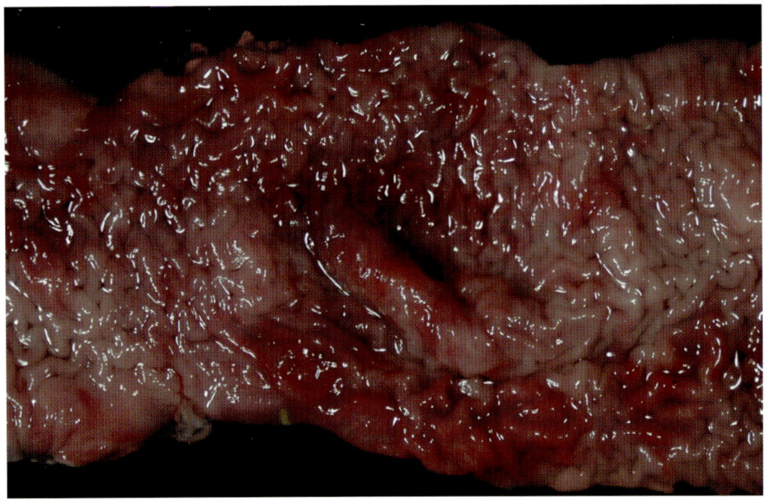

131A Chronic nonproliferative colitis.
Thickened colonic mucosa with irregular red foci. Fattening pig.

131B

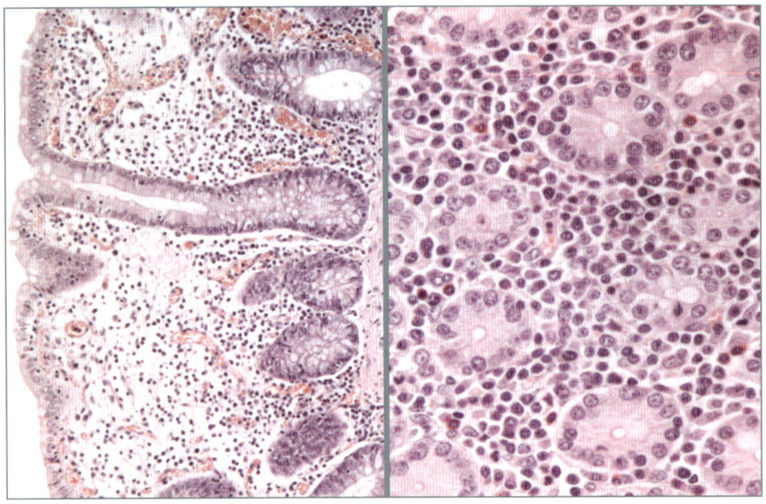

131B Chronic nonproliferative colitis.
Inflammatory cell infiltrate, hyperaemia, and oedema in the lamina propria (left). Predominantly lymphoplasmacytic cell infiltrate in the lamina propria (right). HE.

131C

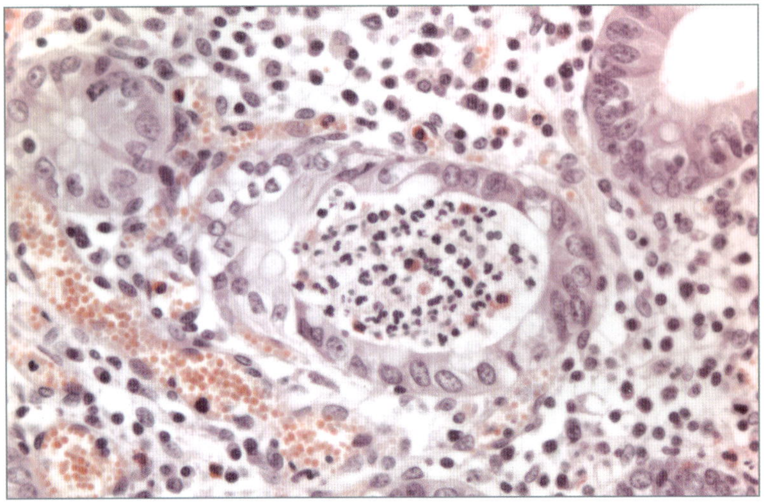

131C Chronic nonproliferative colitis.
Crypt abscess formed by the exudation of neutrophils and eosinophils in the lumen of a dilated crypt. HE.

132A Chronic nonproliferative colitis.

Reddened and unevenly thickened colonic mucosa. Fattening pig.

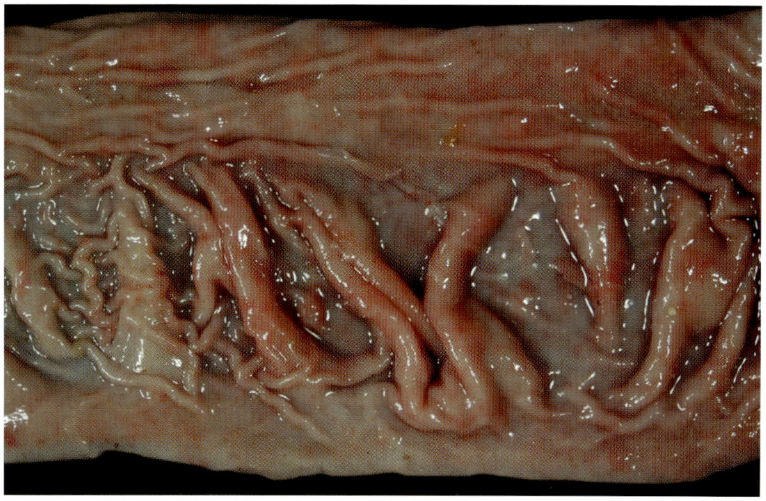

132A

132B Chronic nonproliferative colitis.

Predominantly lymphoplasmacytic inflammatory infiltrate in the lamina propria and formation of crypt abscesses due to granulocyte accumulation in the lumina. HE.

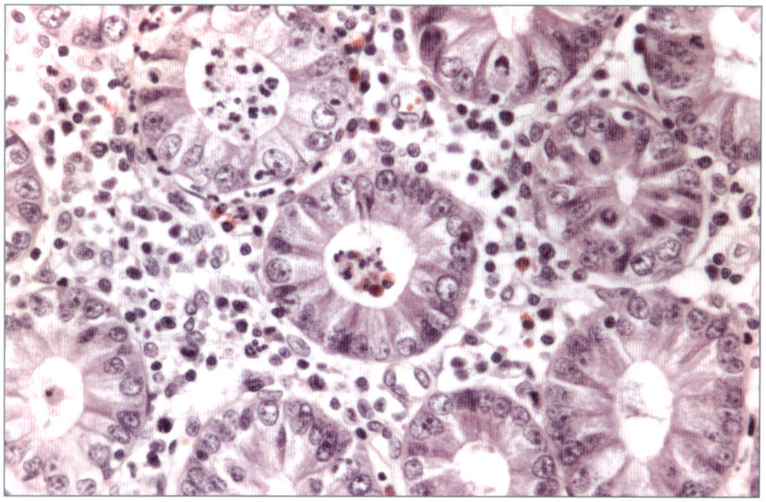

132B

132C Chronic nonproliferative colitis.

Presence of black-stained spiral bacteria on the surface of the mucosa (left) and in the crypts (right). WS.

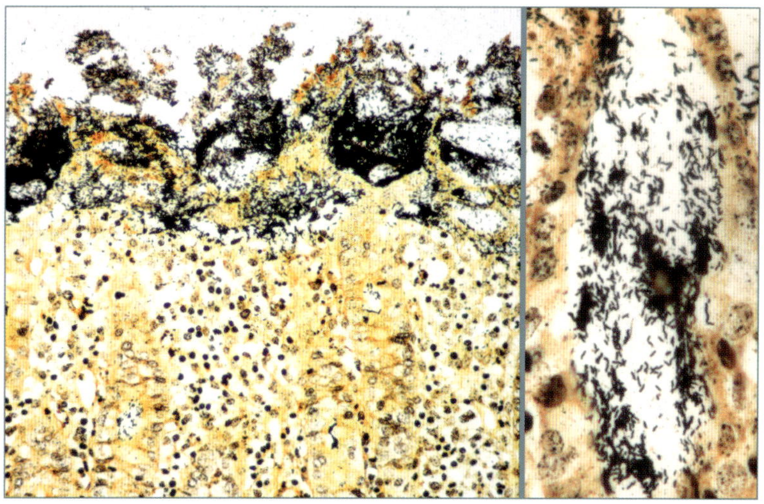

132C

133A

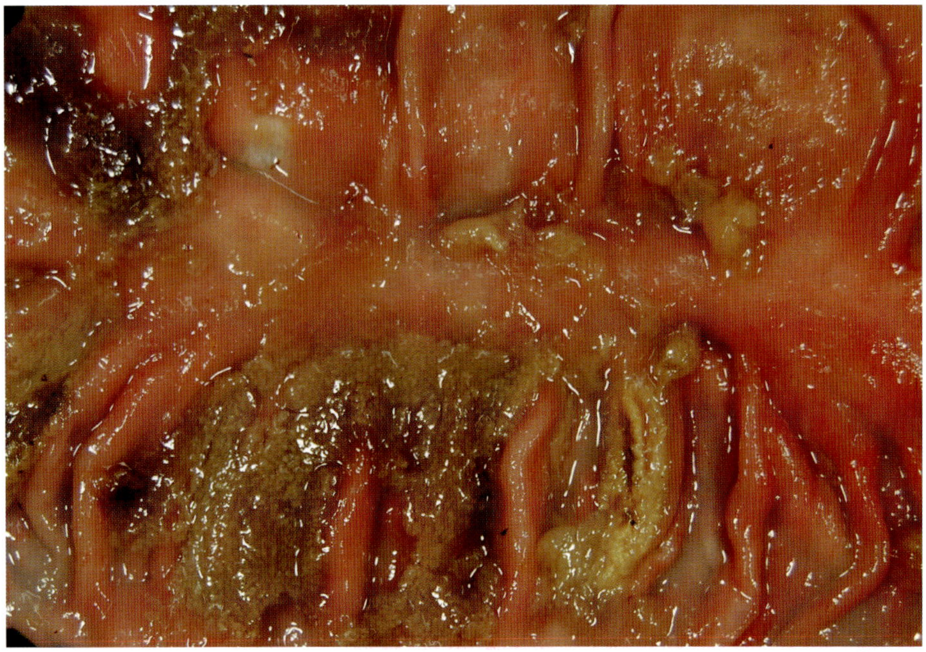

133A

Chronic nonproliferative colitis.

Yellowish-grey plaques of variable extension, composed of mucus and sloughed cells, on the mucosa of the large intestine. Fattening pig.

133B

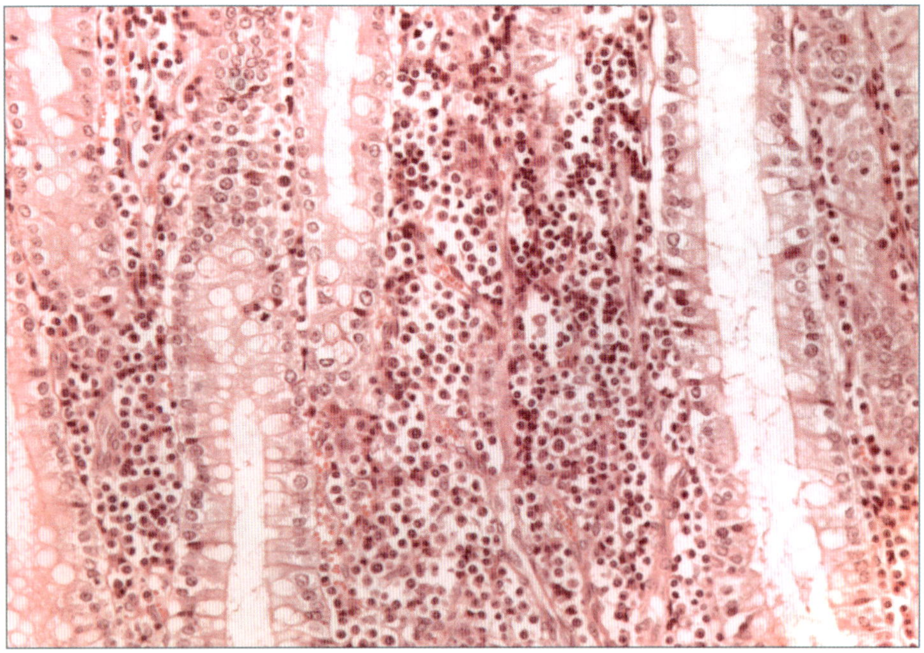

133B

Chronic nonproliferative colitis.

Lymphoplasmacytic infiltrate in the lamina propria. HE.

Chronic nonproliferative colitis is characterised by a predominantly lymphoplasmacytic infiltrate, with epithelial alterations and microabscesses. Some of these alterations, also termed chronic catarrhal colitis or nonspecific colitis, have been linked to the action of potentially infectious agents. In other cases, the aetiopathogenesis is unclear, or attributed to sensitivity to dietary components, with the development of epithelial lesions susceptible to bacterial contamination.

Granulomatous inflammation

This denomination includes chronic intestinal lesions defined by the nature of the cellular inflammatory component, which tend to include diffusely distributed epithelioid cells and multinucleated giant cells.

134A Granulomatous enteritis. Shortening and fusion of the villi, inflammatory cell infiltration of the lamina propria, and elongation of the crypts. HE.

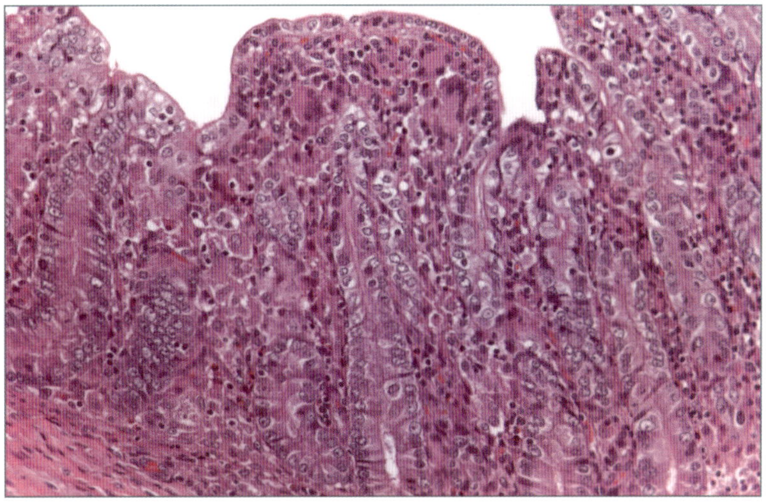

134A

134B Granulomatous enteritis. Lamina propria of the small intestine occupied by a dense inflammatory infiltrate, in which epithelioid macrophages and multinucleated giant cells predominate. Infiltration causing compression of the crypts and distortion and atrophy of the villi. HE.

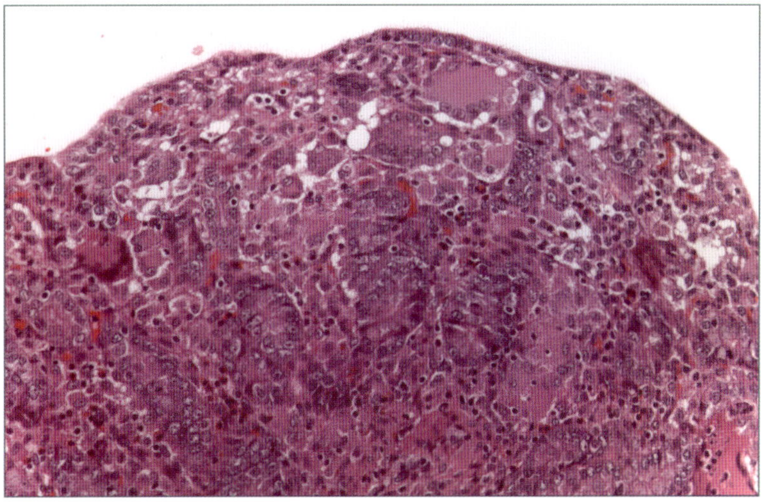

134B

Diffuse forms of granulomatous enterocolitis have been described in infections caused by circovirus and *Mycobacterium avium*. A form of granulomatous enteritis has also been described in pigs with proliferative enteropathy.

Villous atrophy is also associated with chronic intestinal diseases with inflammatory invasion of the lamina propria or proliferation of crypts, usually in weaned animals.

Other forms of inflammation: cystic colitis

135

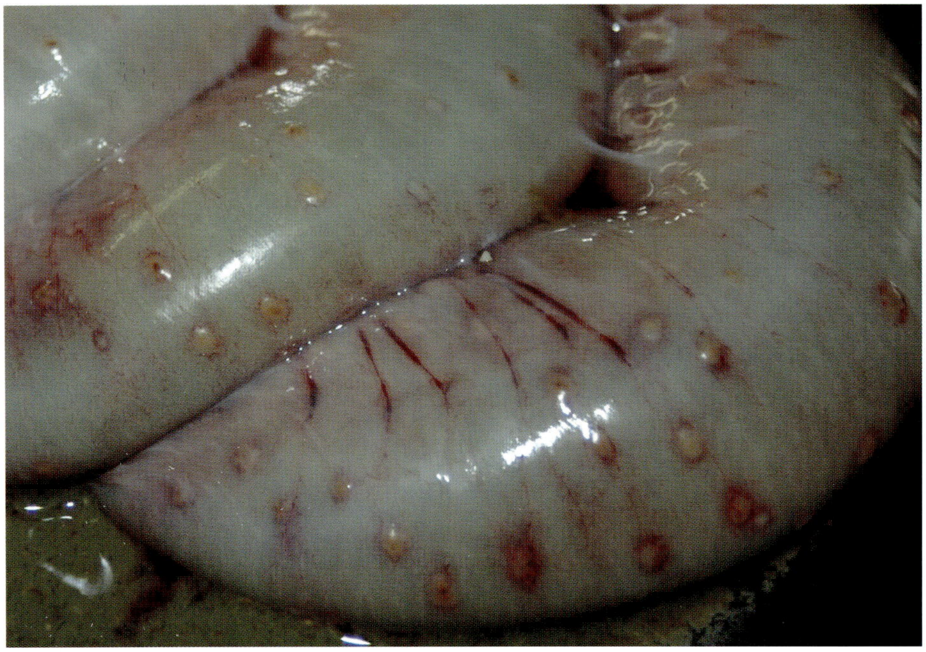

135

Cystic colitis.

Grey nodules, some with reddish borders, visible through the serosa of the large intestine. Fattening pig.

136

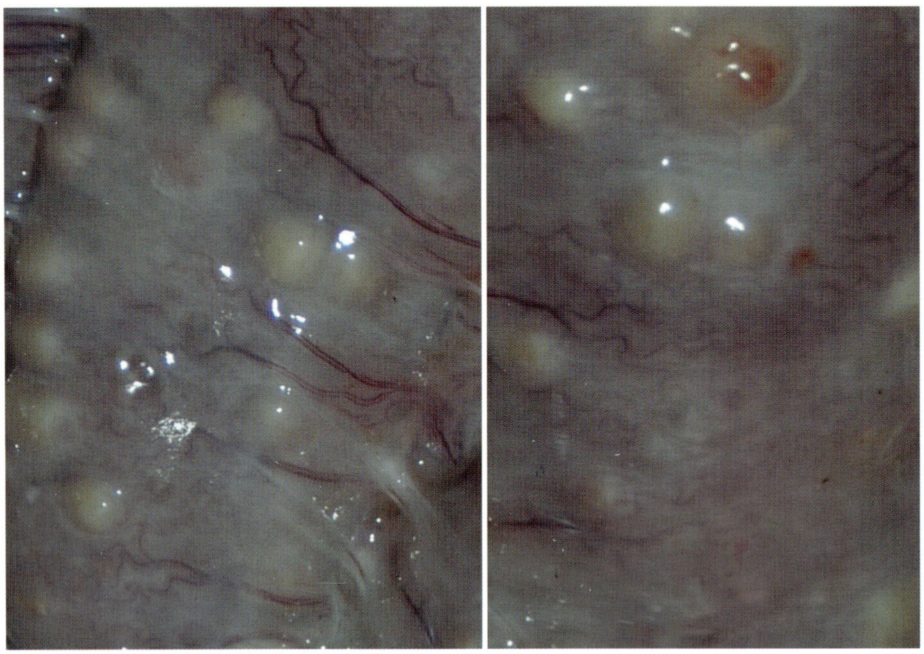

136

Cystic colitis.

Greyish subserosal nodules in different segments of the loops of the colon. Fattening pig.

137A

Cystic colitis.
Whitish nodules projecting through the serosa of the colon (left). Mucosa dotted with small white bumps with a central orifice (right). Fattening pig.

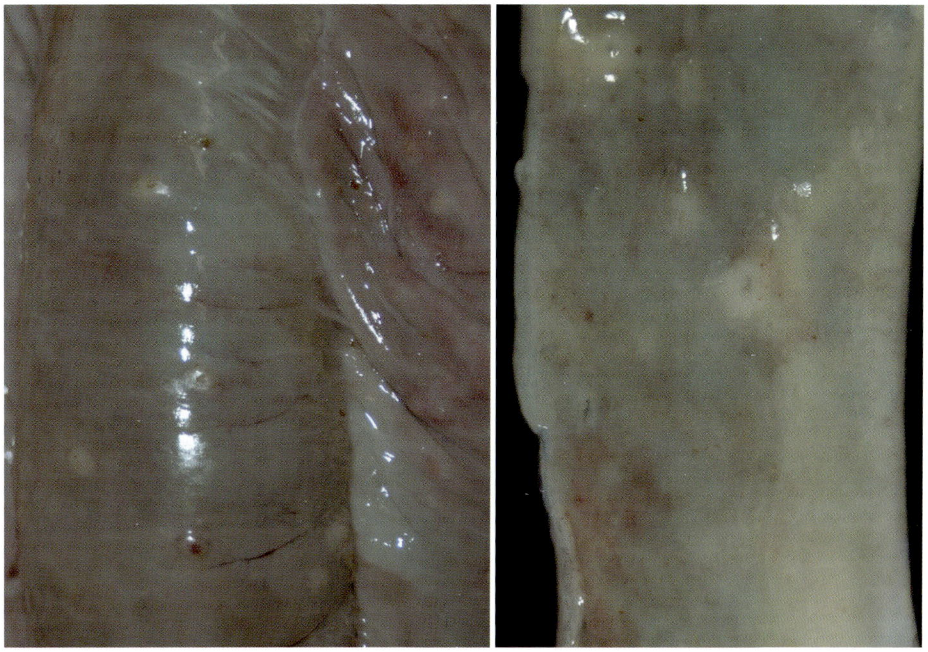

137A

137B

Cystic colitis.
Dilated lymphoglandular complex, filled with mucus, necrotic epithelium, leukocytes, and bacteria. The associated lymphoid tissue is compressed in the periphery and delimited by the epithelium of the cyst wall.

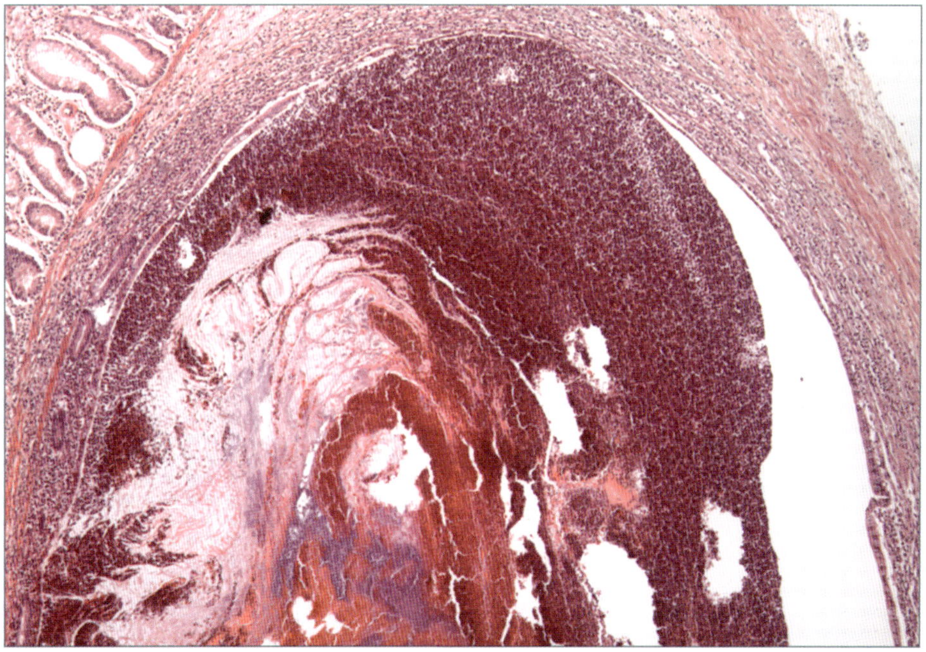

137B

Cystic colitis is not a defined form of inflammation. It is considered a sequela of infectious processes, such as dysentery or salmonellosis, but its significance is unclear. The lesions may be confused with the nodules observed in oesophagostomiasis.

Parasites

138

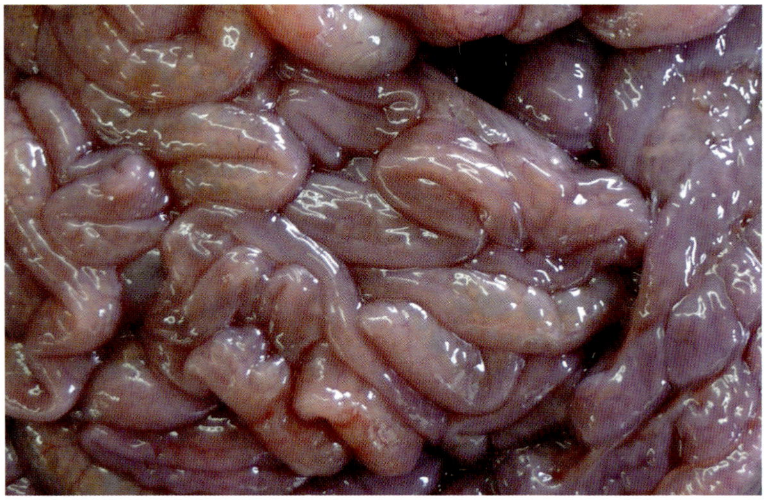

138 **Coccidiosis.**
Flaccid and diffusely dilated loops of the small intestine. Suckling pig.

139A

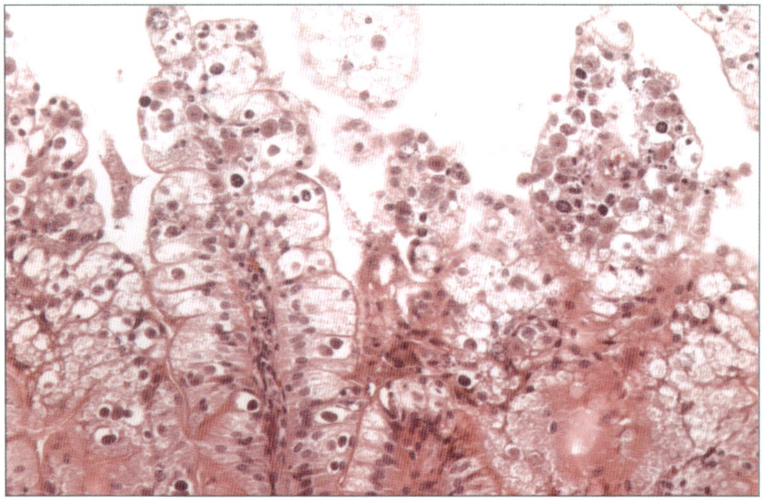

139A **Coccidiosis.**
Retraction of the intestinal villi with vacuolisation of enterocytes caused by intracellular replication of the parasite. HE.

139B

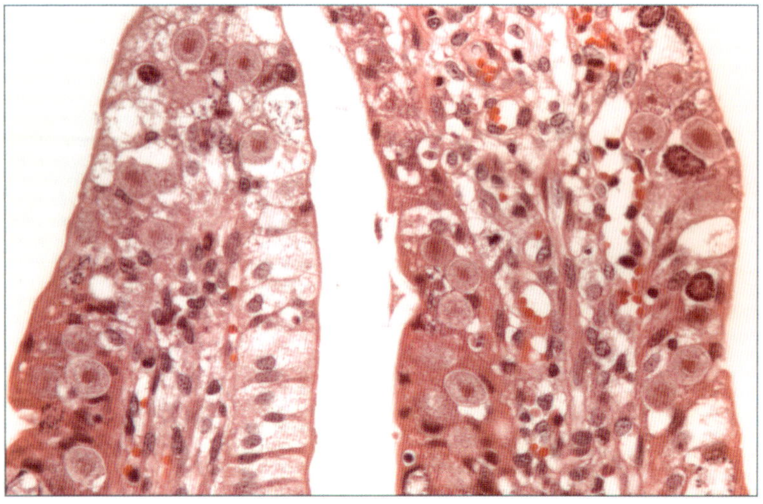

139B **Coccidiosis.**
Epithelial cells of two intestinal villi invaded by intracytoplasmic protozoa in various stages of development. Suckling pig. HE.

140 **Coccidiosis.**
Atrophy and focal necrosis of intestinal villi with overlying pseudomembrane composed of cell debris, leukocytes, and bacterial colonies. Diphtheritic complication of the catarrhal atrophic form. HE.

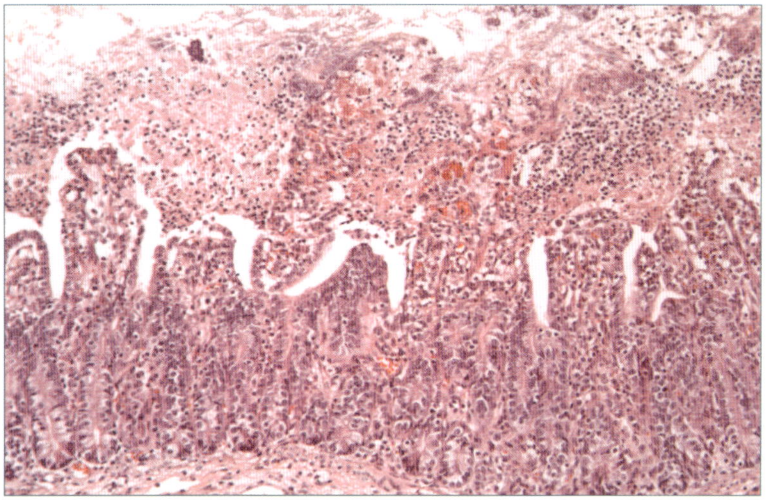
140

141A **Coccidiosis.**
Dilated loops of the small intestine with prominent mesenteric vessels. Suckling pig.

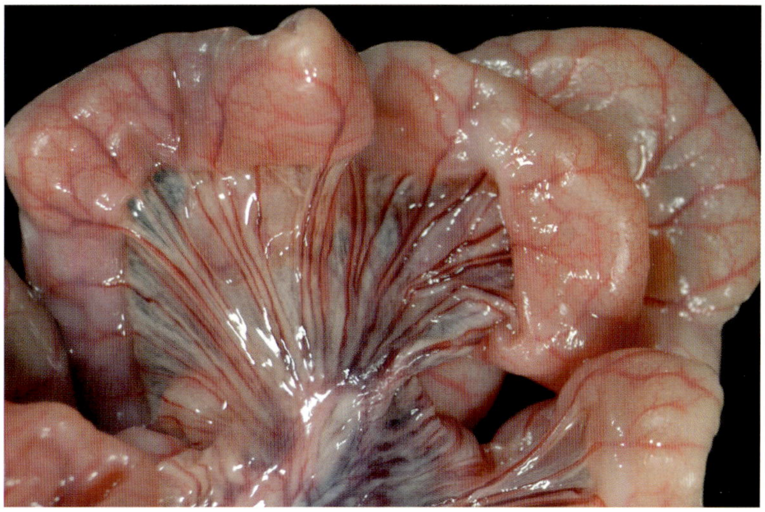
141A

141B **Coccidiosis.**
Atrophy and fusion of intestinal villi with flattening and erosion of superficial enterocytes. HE.

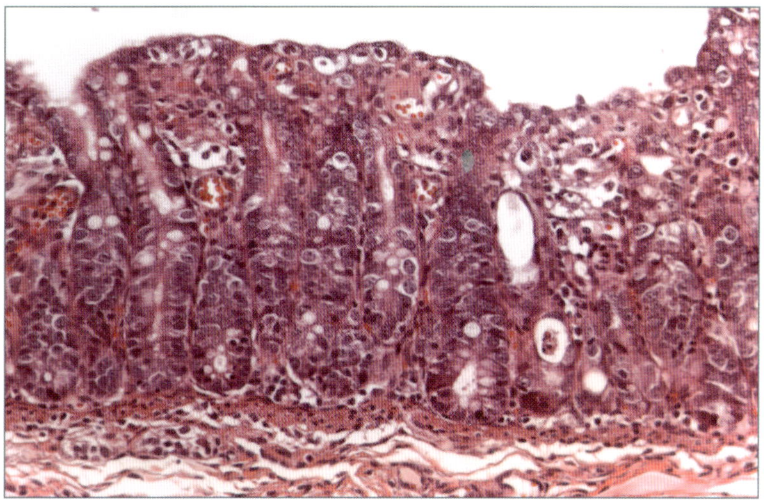
141B

142A

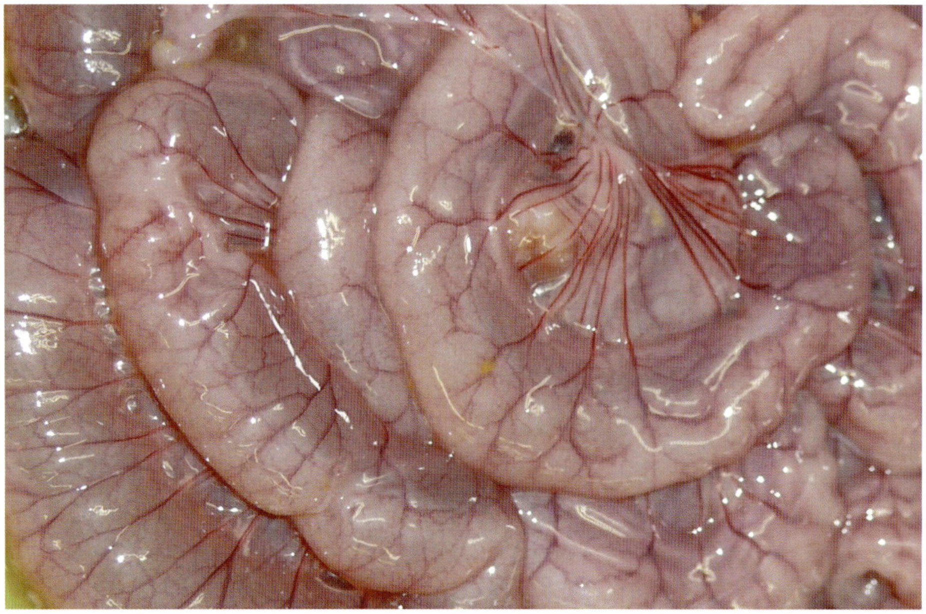

142A

Coccidiosis.

Dilated, flaccid, thin-walled loops of the small intestine, with aqueous content. Suckling pig.

142B

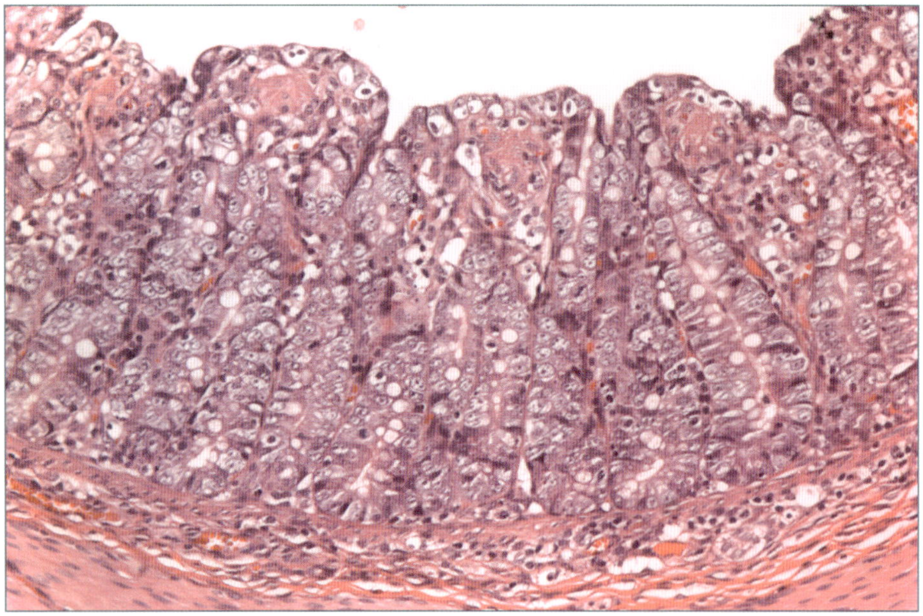

142B

Coccidiosis.

Atrophy and fusion of intestinal villi with developing protozoa in the cytoplasm of the superficial enterocytes, which have been substituted with immature flattened cells. HE.

The most common form of coccidiosis in piglets is caused by *Cystoisospora suis*. Infections caused by this and other species of coccidia are less common in older animals.

143

Cryptosporidiosis.
Basophilic spherule-shaped organisms attached to epithelial cells of the crypts in the large intestine. HE.

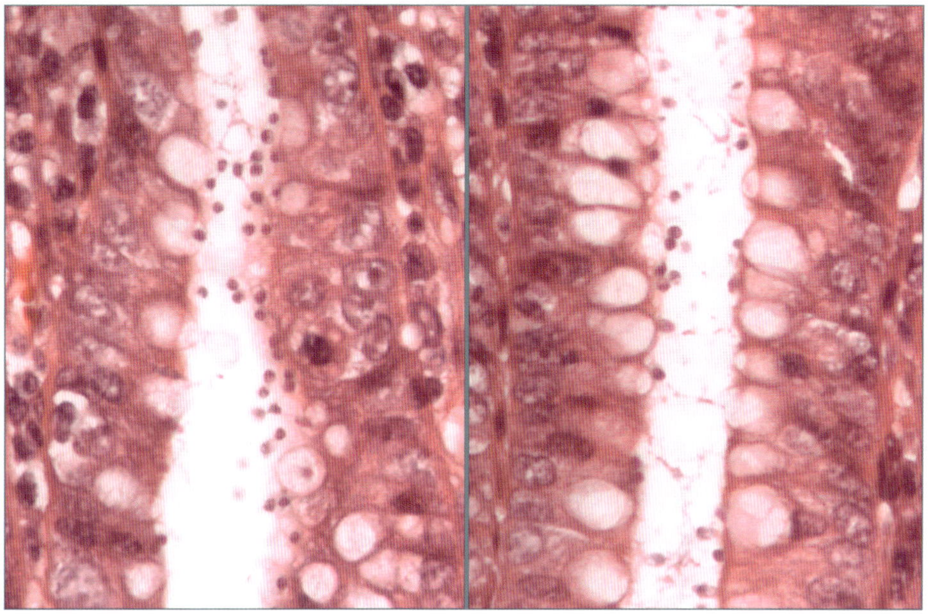

143

Cryptosporidium spp. appears to play a minor role as a primary enteric pathogen. Its action can be exacerbated by the existence of concomitant infections.

144

Trichomonads.
Free protozoan forms in the lumina of the crypts of the large intestine. Weaner pig. HE.

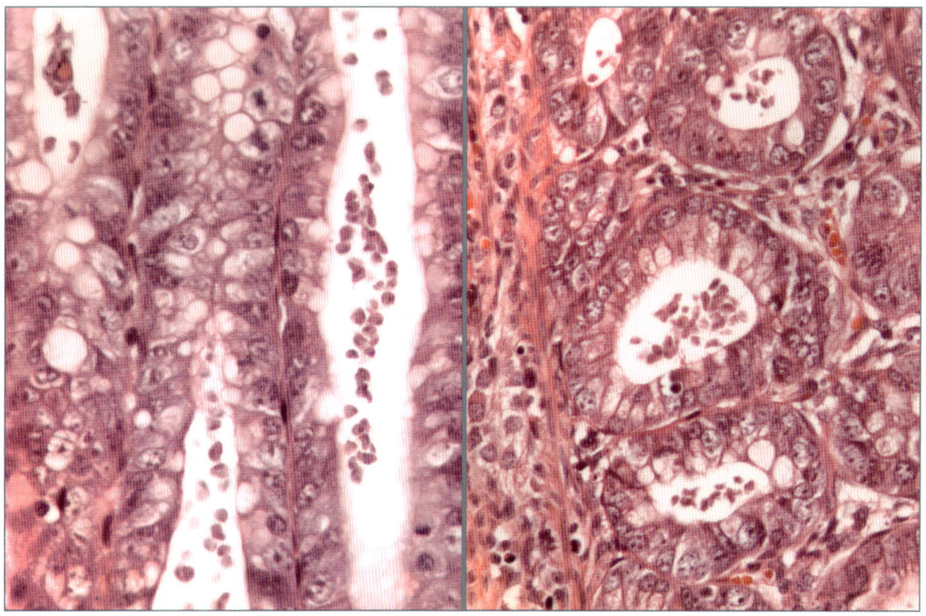

144

145

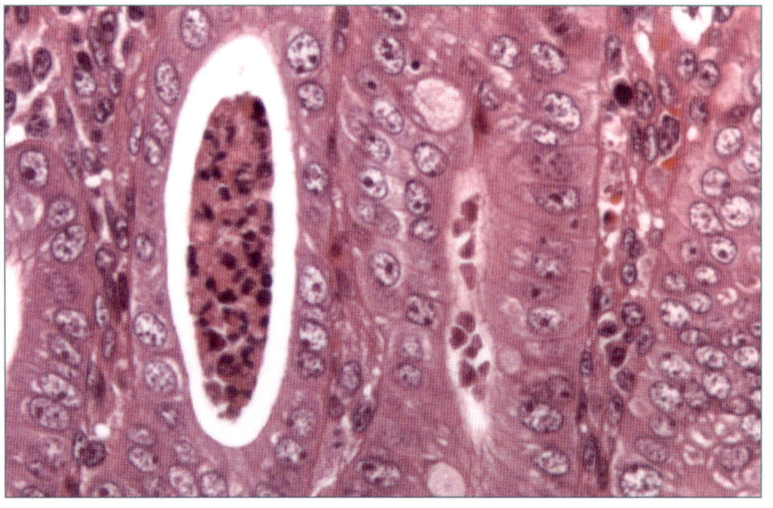

145 Trichomonads.

Free protozoan forms in the crypts of the large intestine and crypt abscess caused by the intraluminal accumulation of inflammatory cells. Weaner pig. HE.

In pigs trichomonads are intestinal parasites with debatable pathogenic action, whose occasional proliferation has been linked to typhlocolitis.

146

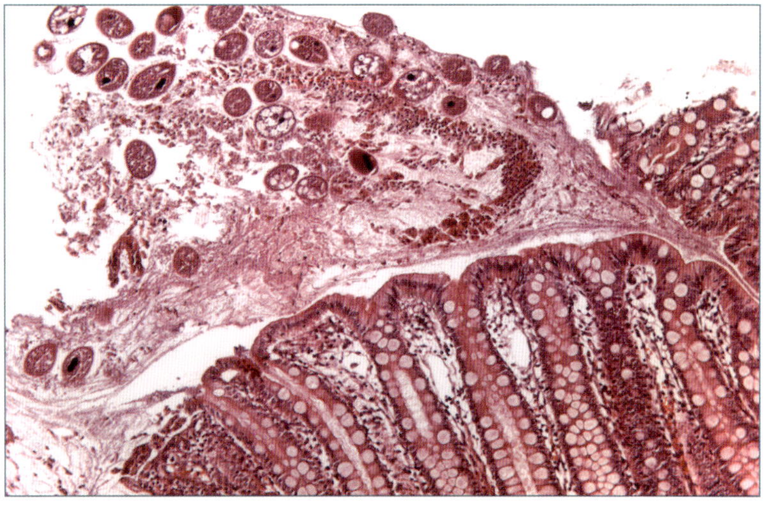

146 Balantidiosis.

Trophozoites in the lumen of the large intestine, recognisable by their size, ovoid shape, and dense nucleus. Weaner pig.

147

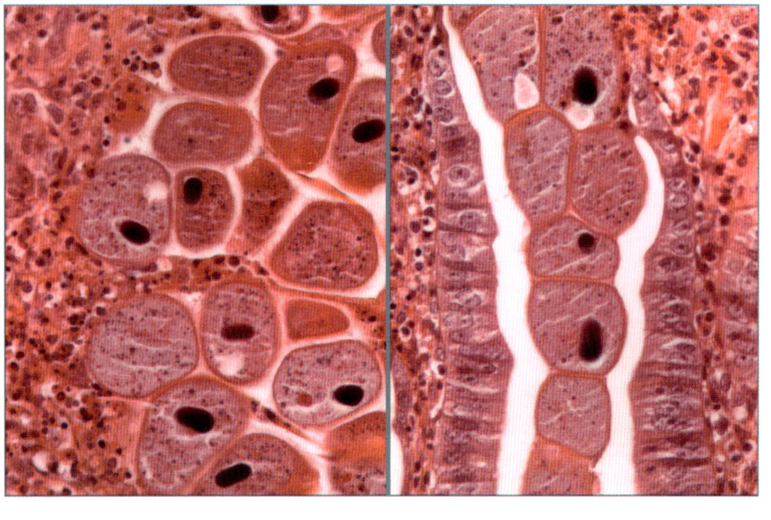

147 Balantidiosis.

Concentration of parasites among necrotic mucosal debris (left) and in the lumen of a crypt (right) in a case of typhlocolitis. Weaner pig. HE.

Balantidium coli is an opportunistic commensal capable of invading the mucosa of the large intestine if the mucosa has been damaged by other diseases such as dysentery or enteric salmonellosis.

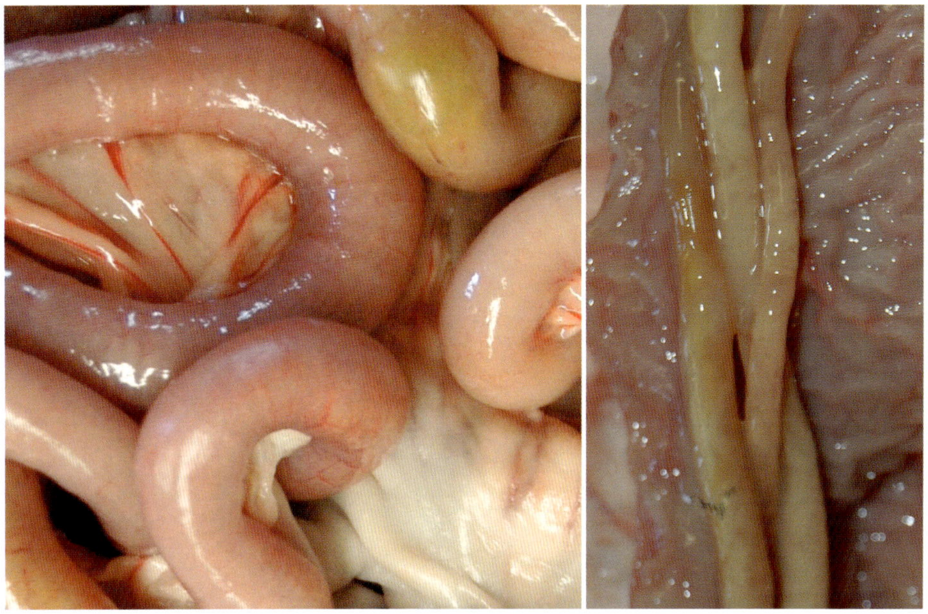

148A

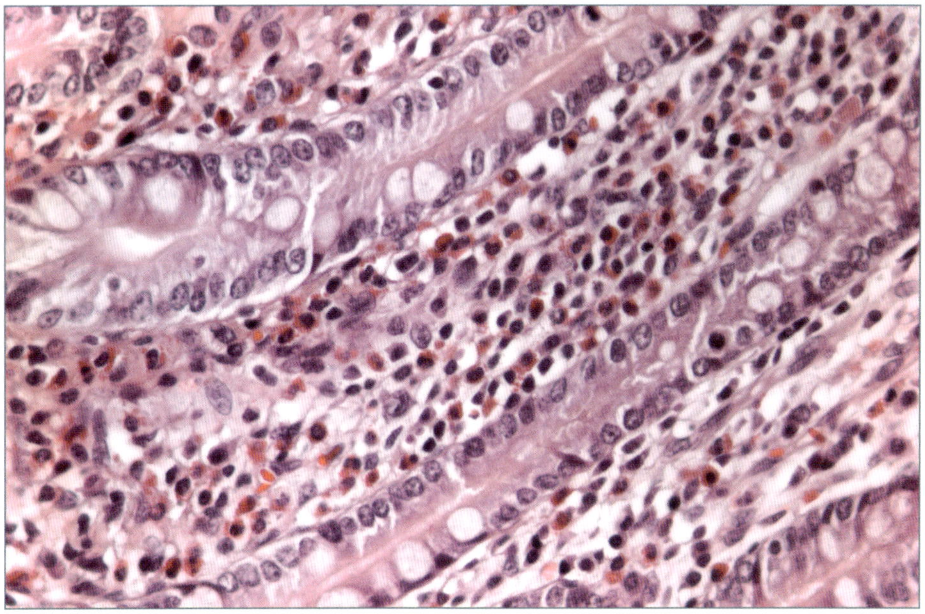

148B

148A Ascariosis.
Swelling of the loops of the small intestine caused by abnormal content, in this case parasites (left). Adult worms on the mucosa of the small intestine (right). Fattening pig.

148B Ascariosis.
Dense leukocyte infiltration in the lamina propria of the intestine with predominance of eosinophils. HE.

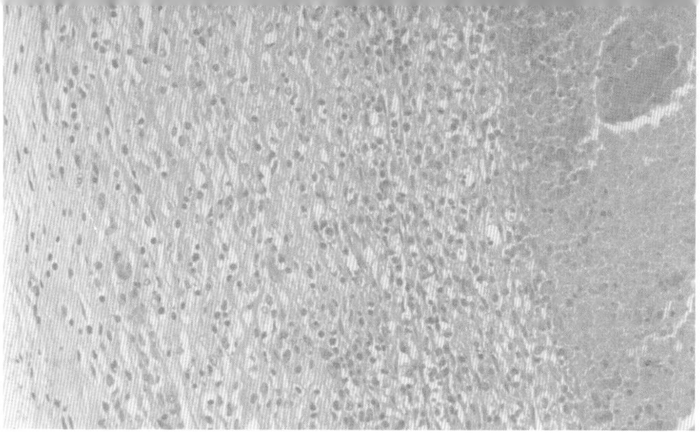

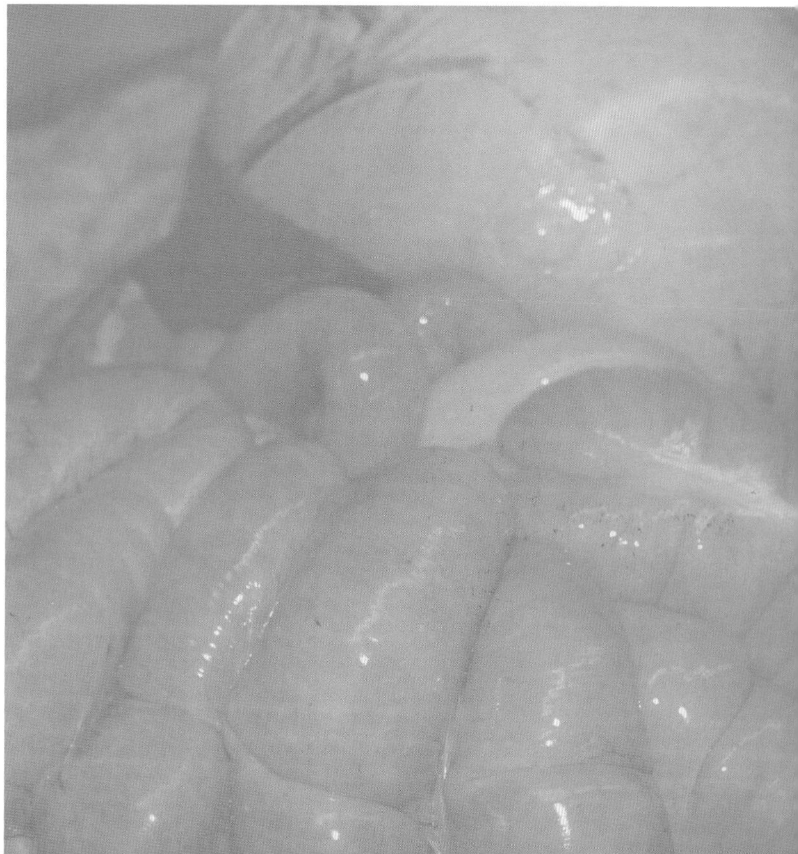

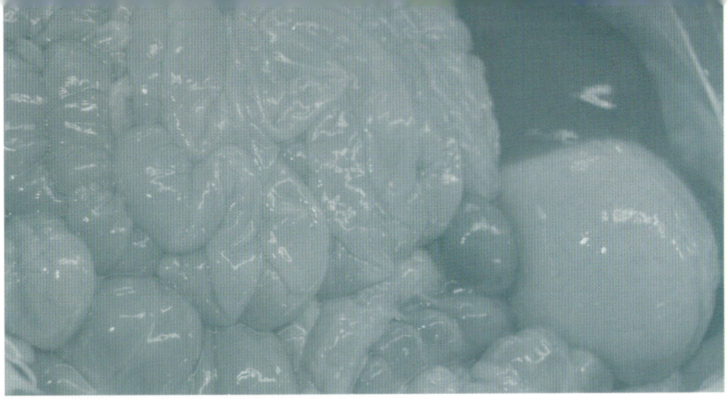

Peritoneum

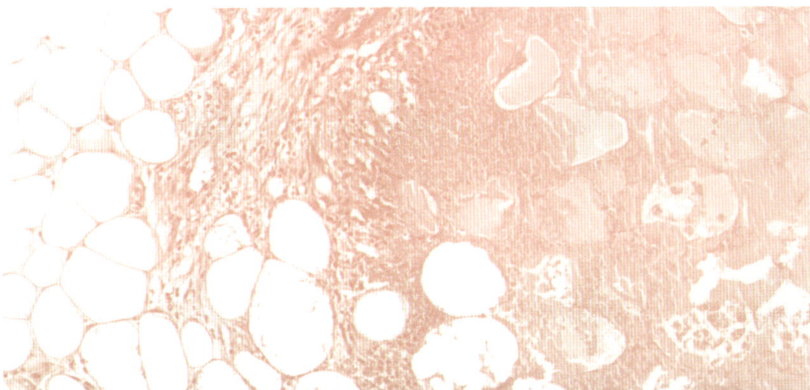

Content alterations

149

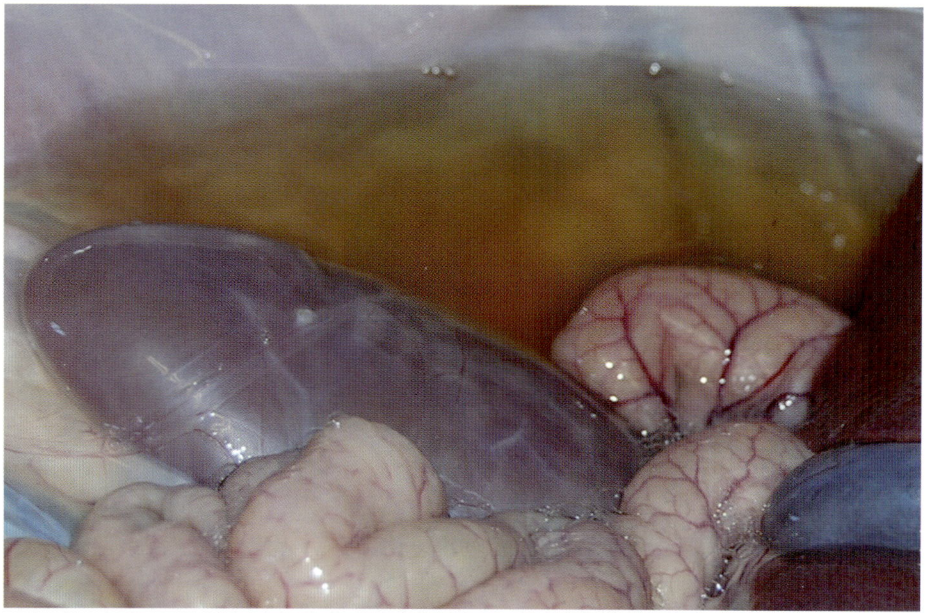

150

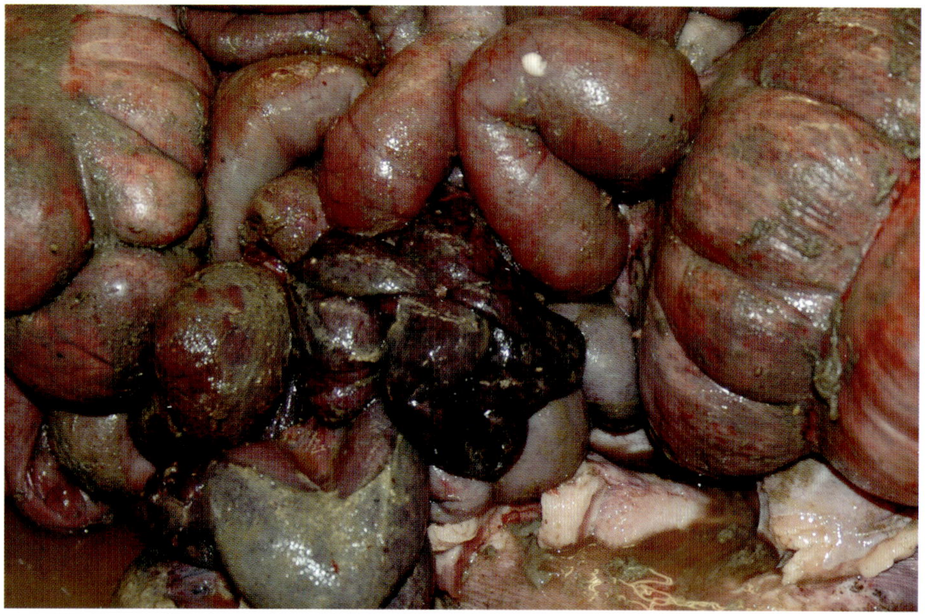

149 **Ascites.**
Accumulation of amber liquid in the abdominal cavity. Fattening pig.

150 **Pathological contents.**
Adherence of the intestinal contents to the serosa with inflammatory reaction associated with perforation. Fattening pig.

The general causes of ascites include cardiac, hepatic, renal, metabolic, and toxic disorders.

Changes in the colour and composition of the peritoneal content are associated with local and systemic infections, haemoperitoneum, metabolic disorders, perforation, and mesenteric torsion.

Hernias

151 **Umbilical hernia.**
Prominent ring and empty hernia sac, with no evident alteration of the parietal peritoneum. Fattening pig.

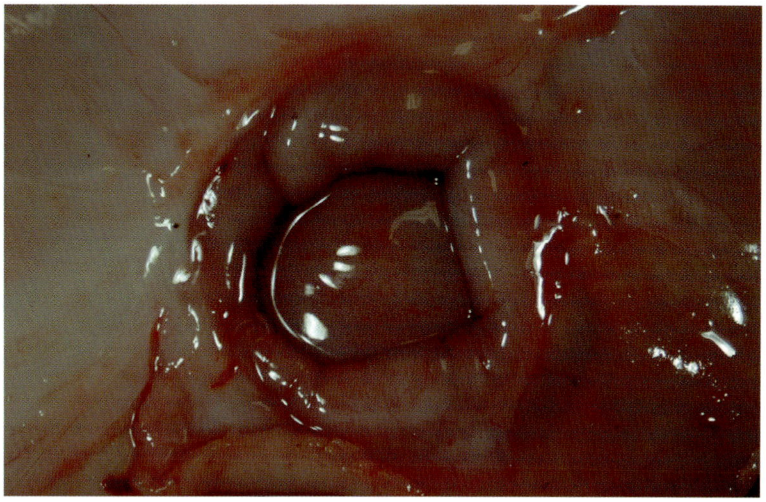

151

152A **Umbilical hernia.**
Thickened and anfractuous hernia sac with the parietal peritoneum covered in yellowish pseudomembranes. Fattening pig.

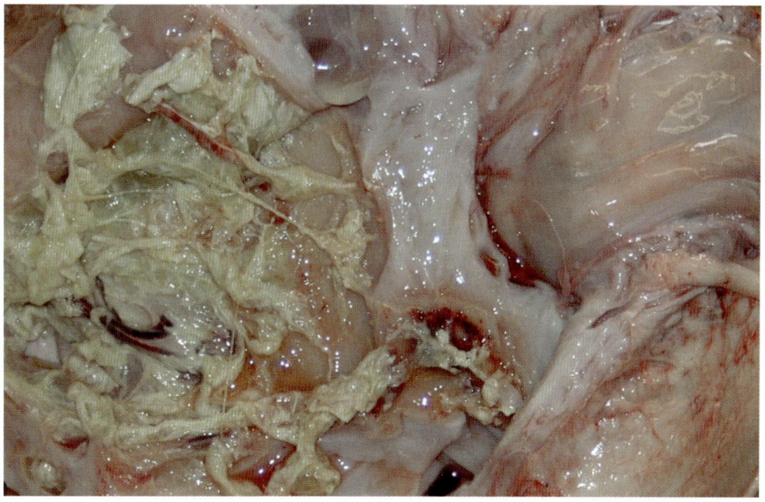

152A

152B **Umbilical hernia.**
Inflammatory reaction of the hernia sac with superficial fibrinous exudate and adjacent fibrosis with inflammatory cell infiltrate.

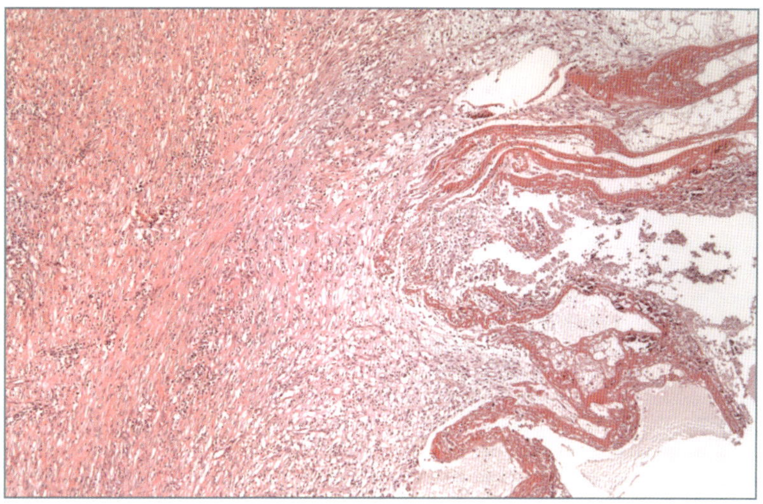

152B

Inflammation

153A

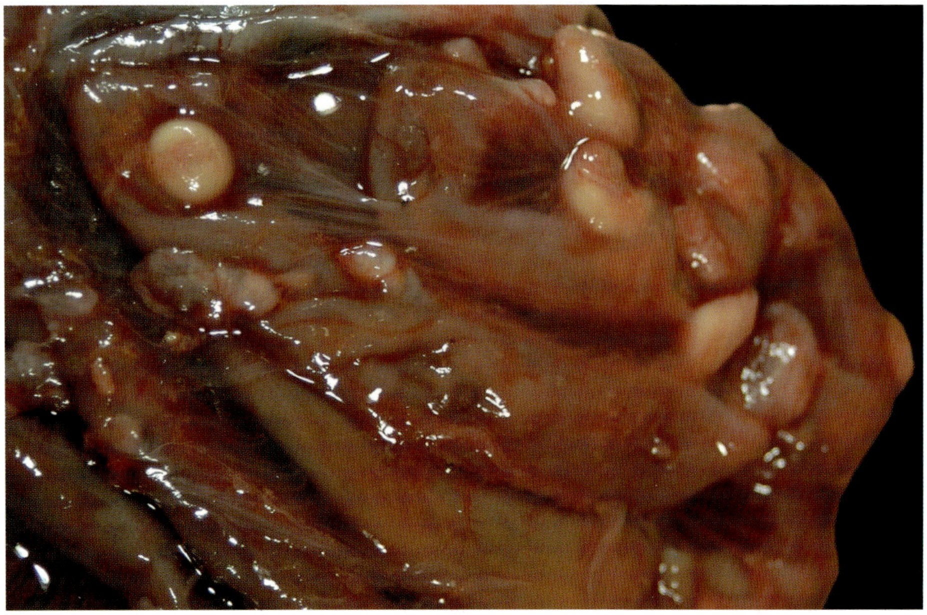

153A

Purulent peritonitis.
Whitish nodules indicating encysted abscesses in the intestinal wall. Weaner pig.

153B

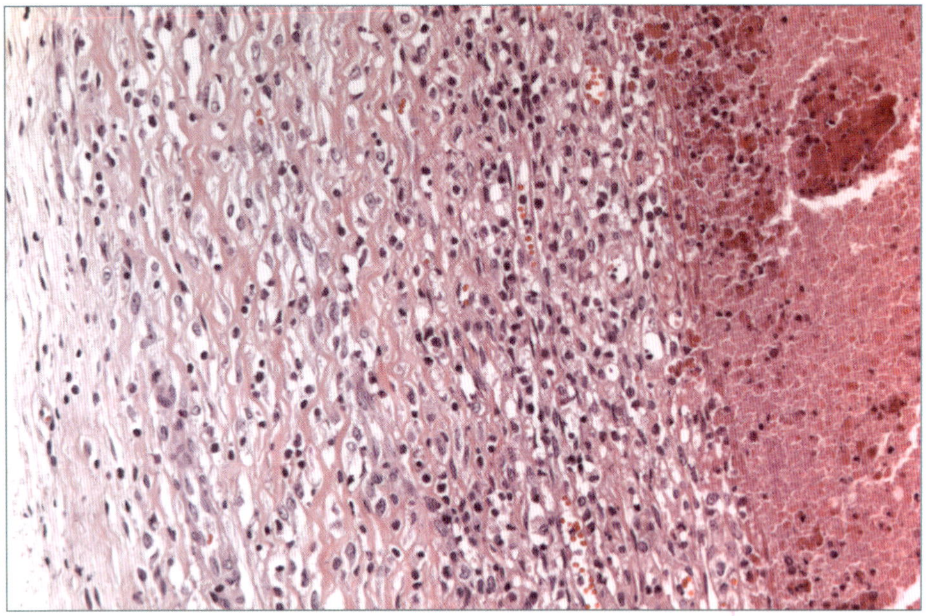

153B

Purulent peritonitis.
Amorphous and acidophilic necrotic focus on the intestinal wall, limited by a connective capsule with inflammatory cell infiltrate. HE.

Abscesses embedded in the peritoneum may be sequelae of infections arising from the extension of castration wounds or umbilical infections.

154 Fibrinous peritonitis.
The surface of the abdominal viscera has a frosted appearance due the presence of inflammatory exudate. Weaner pig.

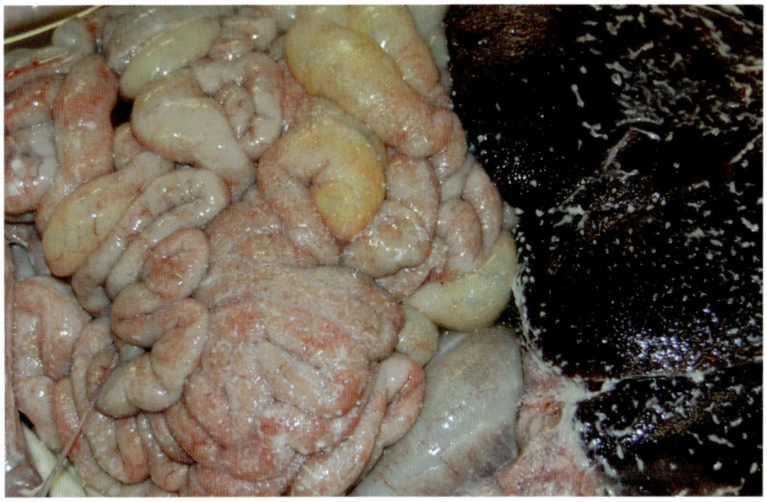
154

155 Fibrinous peritonitis.
Pseudomembranous deposits of variable extension on the parietal peritoneum and the liver capsule. Weaner pig.

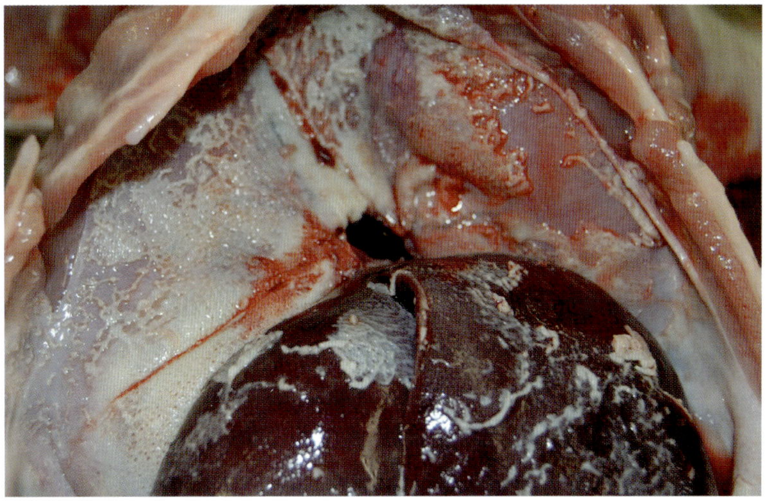
155

156A Fibrinous peritonitis.
Abdominal viscera covered in whitish pseudomembrane in the process of organisation. Weaner pig.

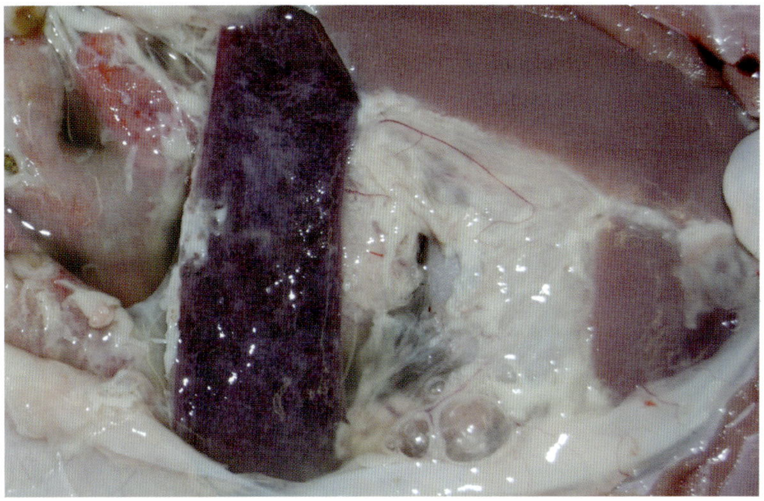
156A

156B

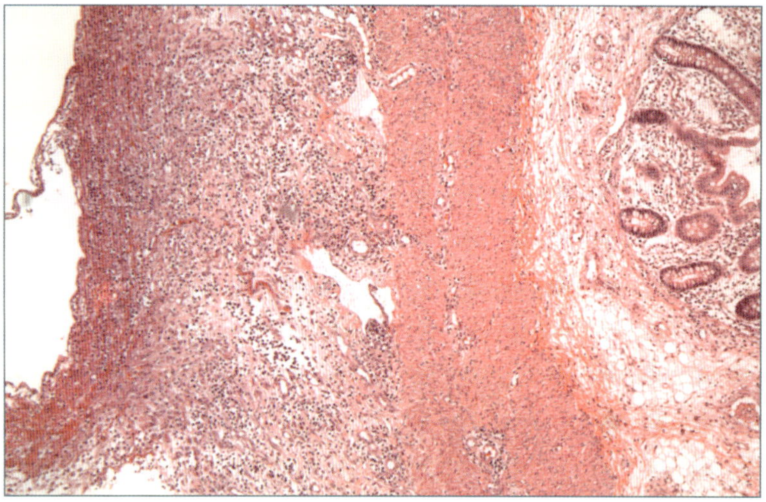

156B **Fibrinous peritonitis.**
Dense pseudomembranous exudate on the intestinal serosa consisting of fibrin strands and inflammatory cells. HE.

156C

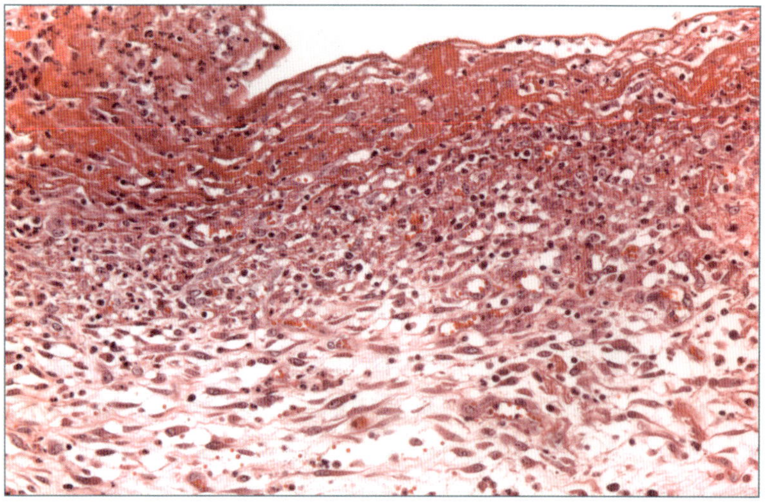

156C **Fibrinous peritonitis.**
Organisation of peritoneal exudate. Proliferation of granulation tissue in the deep portion of the pseudomembrane. HE.

157A

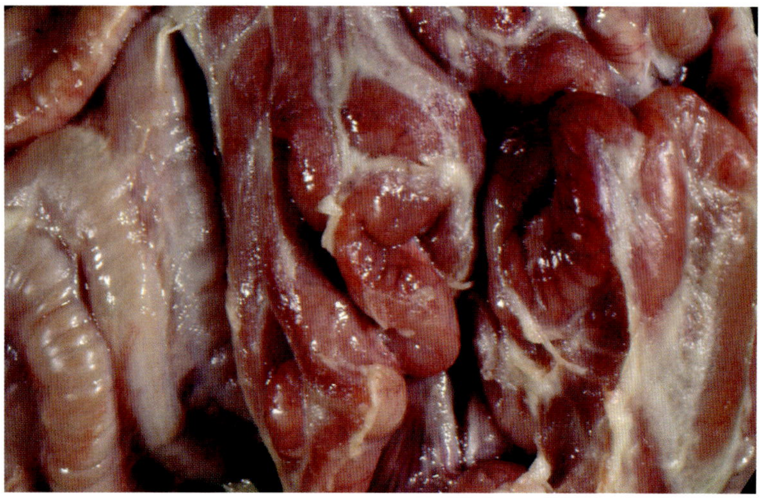

157A **Fibrinous peritonitis.**
Intestinal loops joined by a greyish pseudomembrane in the process of organisation. Weaner pig.

157B **Fibrinous peritonitis.**
Thickening of intestinal serosa caused by a fibrillar acidophilic deposit with numerous leukocytes.

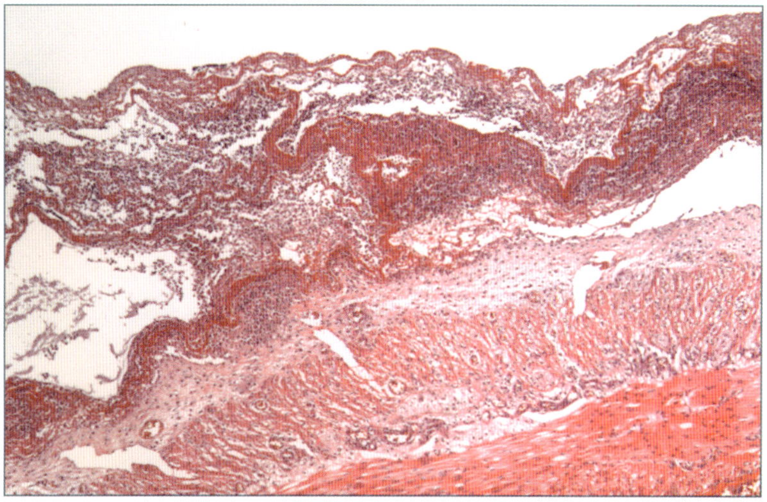

157B

158 **Peritoneal fibrosis.**
Loops of the colon with thickened and wrinkled serosa, caused by the presence of fibrous growths, a sequela of focal peritonitis. Fattening pig.

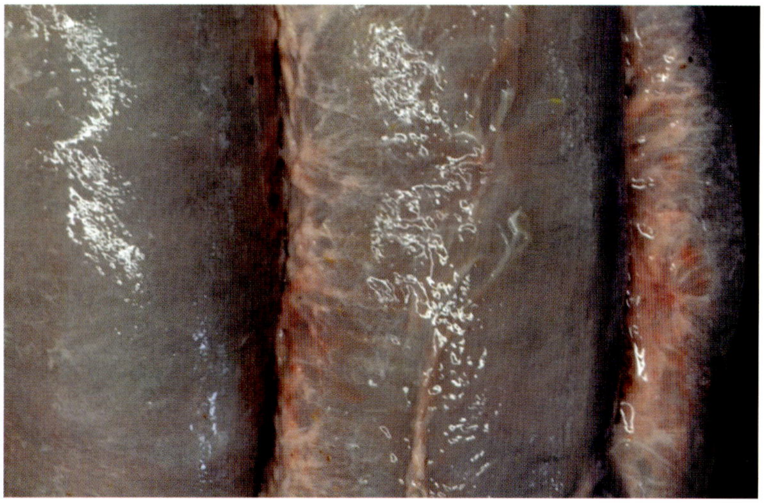

158

Fibrinous peritonitis is associated with enteritis due to *Clostridium perfringens* type C and typhlocolitis due to *Clostridium difficile* in piglets. It is a manifestation of systemic infections caused by *Streptococcus suis*, *Escherichia coli*, *Haemophilus parasuis*, and *Mycoplasma hyorhinis.* It can occur secondary to gastrointestinal perforation and castration wounds. In some processes the serositis and organisation are limited to the colon. Mixed forms are common.

Metabolic disorders

159A

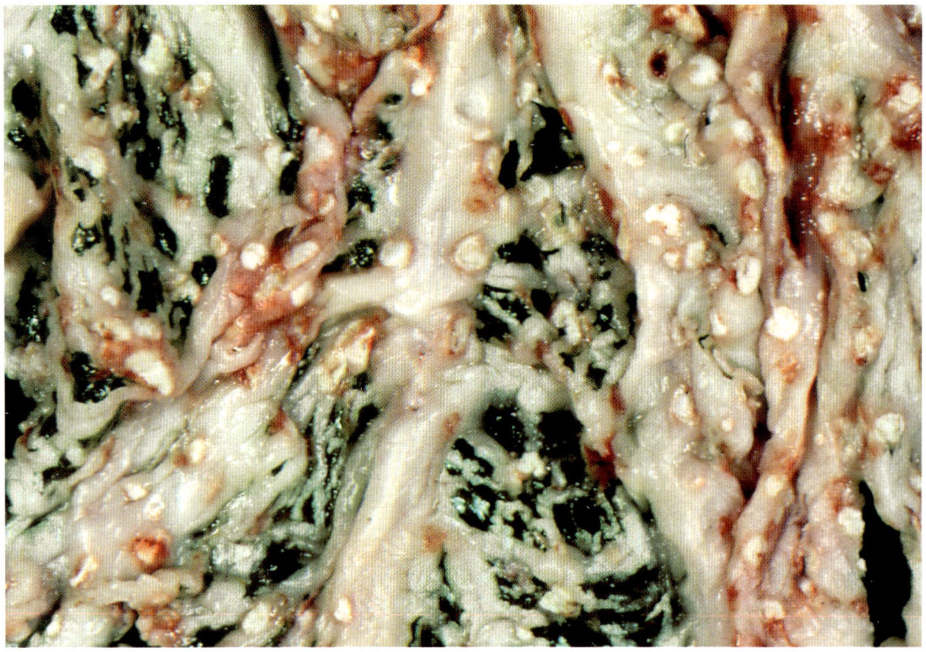

159A

Fat necrosis.
Whitish, desiccated-looking multifocal deposits, with a reddish margin, located in the omentum. Fattening pig.

159B

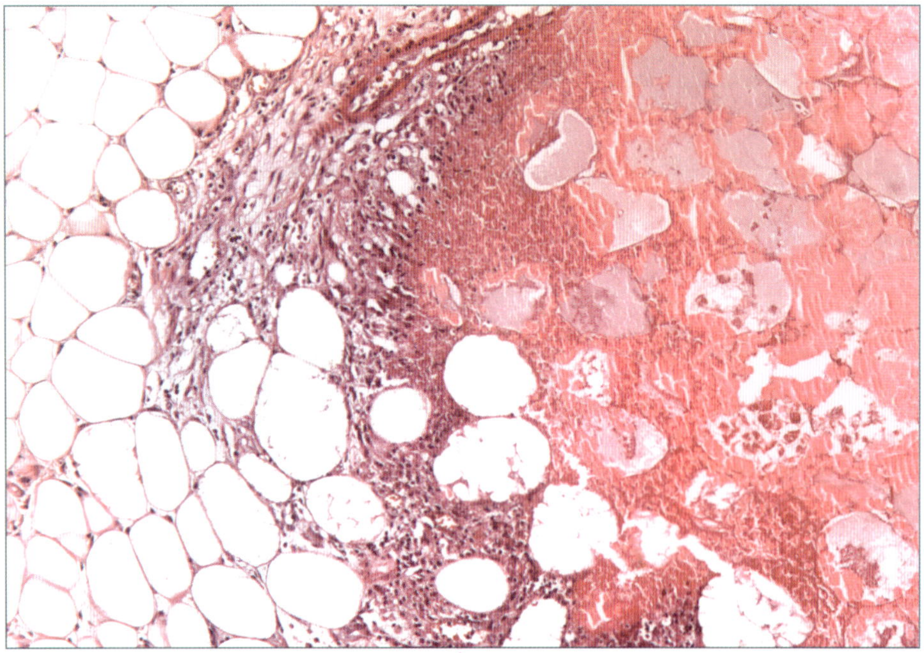

159B

Fat necrosis.
Focus of large fat cells with poorly defined borders, delimited from the adjacent adipose tissue by an inflammatory cell infiltrate. HE.

Among other causes, abdominal fat necrosis is attributed to the release of pancreatic enzymes in response to inflammation, pressure, or trauma.

Parasites

160

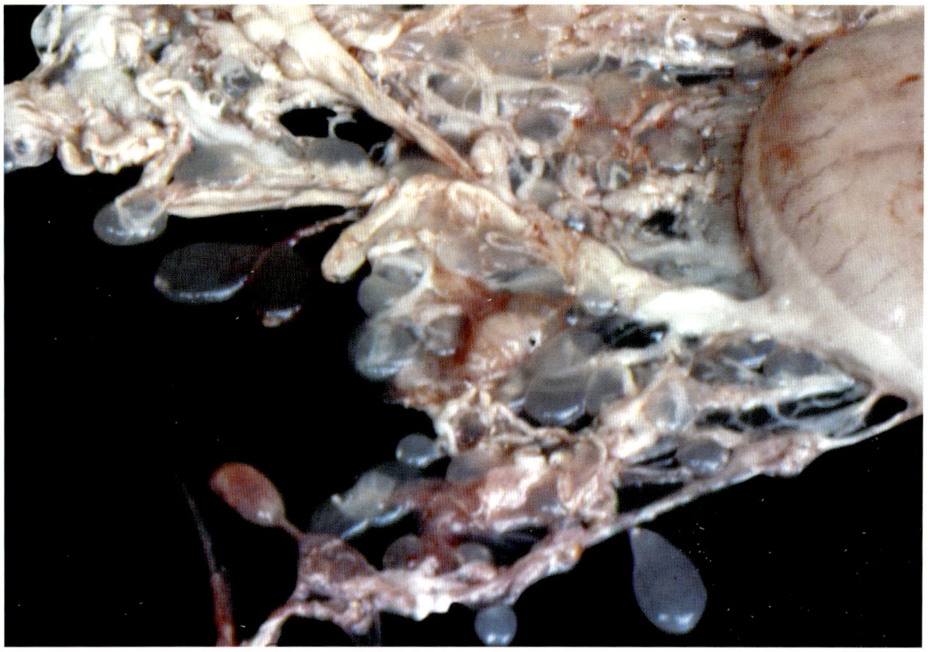

160

Visceral cysticercosis.
Translucent vesicles in the omentum, isolated or grouped in small clusters.
Fattening pig.

161

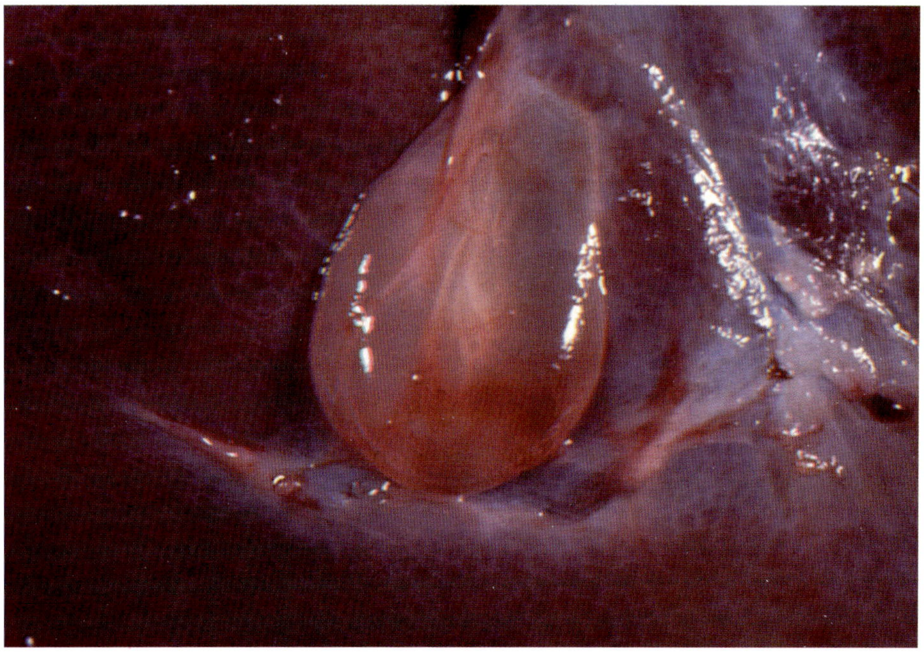

161

Visceral cysticercosis.
Thin-walled vesicle, through which the invaginated scolex can be observed, adhered to the liver surface.
Fattening pig.

Published by Servet editorial - Grupo Asís Biomedia S.L.